Radical Acts of Love

Radical Acts of Love

Twenty Conversations to
Inspire Hope at the End of Life

JANIE BROWN

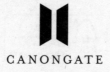

CANONGATE

This paperback edition first published in Great Britain and the USA in 2021
by Canongate Books

Distributed in the USA by Publishers Group West

First published in Great Britain in 2020 by Canongate Books Ltd,
14 High Street, Edinburgh EH1 1TE

canongate.co.uk

1

British Library Cataloguing-in-Publication Data
A catalogue record for this book is available on
request from the British Library

ISBN 978 1 78689 9 033

Typeset in Mrs Eaves by Palimpsest Book Production Ltd,
Falkirk, Stirlingshire

Printed and bound in Great Britain by Clays Ltd, Elcograf S.p.A.

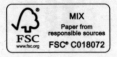

MIX
Paper from
responsible sources
FSC® C018072
FSC www.fsc.org

FOR KIRSTEN,
WHO INSPIRED ME TO WRITE

AND FOR ALL THE OTHER PEOPLE
IN THIS BOOK
WHO ALSO GRACED ME WITH
THEIR LIVES

'If you would indeed behold the spirit of death,
open your heart wide unto the body of life.'

— 'DEATH POEM XXVII' BY KHALIL GIBRAN

'He, too, has been changed in his turn,
Transformed utterly:
A terrible beauty is born.'

— 'EASTER, 1916' BY W.B. YEATS

Contents

III. HEALING THE TROUBLED HEART

IV. SURRENDERING TO THE SPACIOUS HEART

Preface

Gran was the first person I saw die. I was nineteen years old and she was eighty-one. She was my father's mother and she lived with our family for the last couple of years of her life, in a small cottage attached to the old sandstone house my three siblings and I were raised in, just outside Glasgow. Gran died of oesophageal cancer, more common in those days because of the heavy cigarette-smoking combined with her daily tipples of whisky. I remember following Mum into Gran's bright white bedroom and watching over her shoulder as she washed my grandmother and changed the soiled sheets. I wanted to help her care for Gran but I felt frozen, unsure what to do, even though I had worked in hospitals for two summers by that time. Gran was my kin, not a patient. That made a difference then.

I don't remember being afraid of death, rather just curious about the unusual smells in the room and the fact that she coughed a lot and didn't talk much. Mum made it okay. She didn't seem afraid either, just busy. She had been a nurse too, which must have helped her know what to do. There were no long heartfelt conversations at Gran's bedside, nor long bucket lists of activities to be accomplished. There was just the work of dying – for my gran, the patient, and for my mum, the caregiver.

I learned then that most deaths are natural. Not easy, but not necessarily scary; nor traumatic or over-medicalised; not romantic nor glorified. Death is most often ordinary and manageable, acceptable but deeply sad. The majority of old people, like my grandmother, died at home in those days before it was commonplace to be admitted to a hospital, or hospice, for the last days or weeks of life.

Most people now under sixty have never seen a person die, so have become deeply fearful about death; both their own, and the deaths of their beloved others. They have had no role models to show them how to care for a dying person, and therefore no confidence in being able to do so. My hope is that the baby boomer cohort who pushed for the return of the midwives to de-medicalise birth will also be instrumental in reclaiming the death process. This book is my contribution to the re-empowering of all of us to take charge of our lives and our deaths, remembering that we know how to die, just as we knew how to come into this world. We also know how to heal, and how to settle our lives as best we can before we die. In my view, this is the greatest gift we could give our loved ones: to be prepared and open and accepting when the time comes for us to leave this world.

My first summer job was at the Glasgow Sick Children's Hospital, working as a nurses' aide on the orthopaedic floor. Frustrated Glaswegian kids with broken bones, strung up on traction, yelled at me to fetch things and made fun of me if I messed up. Even though their demands intimidated me, at sixteen I loved the feeling of being helpful. The following summer I worked in a psychiatric hospital for the elderly where many patients had been hospitalised for thirty or forty years. I remember an ancient, scary woman who shuffled along behind me everywhere I went, and stared at my every move like an owl contemplating her prey. At a young age, I was compelled to try to understand the brokenness of humanity.

When I enrolled at St Andrews University, I planned to study geography. I had always loved maps, and still do, but in my third year I declared a major in psychology. The study of human behaviour trumped my interest in topography. I graduated in 1980 with an MA in Psychology, and the following spring I became a student again, studying nursing at the Royal Infirmary in Edinburgh. I wanted to travel and work at a job that was in demand across countries and cultures, and to find a way to make a difference in the world.

I was twenty-two and had been a student nurse for six months when I was assigned to care for a man in his forties dying of leukaemia. He had just been moved from the main ward, with its fifteen beds down either side, to one of only two private rooms. Standing nervously outside his room that evening, as my heart hammered against my ribcage, I thought about what I would say:

Good evening Mr Stevens, I'm Nurse Brown, here for the night shift. How are you feeling?

I wasn't sure that my experience with Gran or nursing school had prepared me for this.

I took a deep breath and knocked softly on Mr Stevens' door. A stronger voice than I was expecting said, 'Come in.'

The darkened room enveloped me as I stepped in, my eyes taking a few moments to adjust.

'Hello, you must be my nurse for tonight. Just call me Jack, will you? All this formality – not much use for it at this stage of my life.'

'Good evening. I'm Nurse Brown,' I said. I wasn't allowed to tell patients my first name or call them by theirs, though I always wanted to. His baldness struck me, as did the dark circles under his eyes.

The photograph by Jack's bed caught my eye. A family shot, taken on a windy day somewhere on the coast. The woman's dark hair was blown across most of her face; she had a joy about her. Two children: a boy about eight years old, a cheeky face, a red-head; and a little girl, perhaps five, holding on to a soggy-looking cracker, a shy glance at the camera.

'The summer holidays?' I asked, glad for the opener.

'Just this past summer, on Islay,' Jack replied. 'Bitter wind, but we love it there, been going since Alistair was a baby. Won't be any more of those holidays now, at least not with the four of us.'

'Mmm,' I said, at a loss for words. Tears threatened, but *not now.* I bustled around the room, straightened the pile of paperbacks, folded the *Guardian* and popped a few scrunched tissues into the paper rubbish bag taped to the edge of the tabletop.

'Shall I refill your ice water?' I asked.

'Thanks. The painkillers make me unbelievably thirsty.'

I picked up the Styrofoam cup, glad for the excuse to step out of the room. As I stood at the ice machine, the clatter of the cubes dropping into the empty cup soothed me with its ordinariness.

Although I felt awkward and incompetent to help Jack with his vast sadness and fears about dying, over the next few days he put me at ease by talking openly about his feelings. He described the guilt he felt about leaving his children and his wife, even though he knew cancer wasn't his fault, and he worried about the pain his death would cause them.

With Jack, I learned that it was not my responsibility to take away his sorrow and worry, but more to offer a soft place of caring for his feelings to land. I found that if I mostly listened and spoke rarely, Jack talked himself through his feelings until he finally ran out of words, and a deep quiet wrapped around us. The space between us seemed to connect us both to something larger, a perspective that I know now, more than thirty years later, can be deeply comforting in those moments when words make little sense.

Jack's openness and vulnerability inspired me to learn more about how people live with dying, and how healthcare professionals can support people better through emotionally and spiritually difficult times. He taught me that a quiet, steady, non-judgemental presence – and a deep faith in the person's ability to find his or her own way to navigate life's end – is the cornerstone of any useful caregiving.

It feels to me that this quality of presence originates and emanates from the heart; not the physical organ, but an emotional centre where a particular sensation gathers – perhaps it is love or compassion – generated in response to another's suffering. This connection through suffering can create a feeling of spaciousness or wholeness between two people that I believe is the potential healing space.

The experience with Jack propelled me to seek a deeper understanding of how to create the conditions whereby this wholeness can be evoked. I will always be grateful to him for my initiation into the work that has become central to my life.

A few years later, when I was twenty-six, I wanted to spend a year living and working in a different country, so I went to Canada. A twelve-month stay turned into one of over thirty years. I worked as an oncology nurse in Vancouver for ten years, and it was during that time that both my love for the work and my dissatisfaction with the system within which I practised grew. I became frustrated with a healthcare model that focused more on treating the disease of cancer than the person with the illness. I wanted more time to attend to the heart and the spirit of a person, and their loved ones.

I also became disheartened with a culture that was no longer empowered in its relationship with death.

I saw how afraid healthcare professionals and many oncologists were discussing death with their patients, let alone providing tools to help them address their fears and worries.

In retrospect, I realise I was also struggling to handle the pain of my chosen vocation. I didn't know how to grieve the people I cared for who had died and I didn't know who, or what, to rage at. I felt responsible for what happened to a person, and what didn't happen. I saw cancer as the enemy, and I joined in the fight. Standing up for what we believe in is the daily practice of oncology nurses, but I had yet to learn how to do that *and* keep my heart open.

I wanted to change myself and change the system.

After returning to university and completing my MSc in Nursing, I took a full-time position as a clinical nurse specialist, which allowed me to continue to work directly with patients, families and nurses in a counselling role. I have the utmost respect for nurses who become educators, researchers and administrators, but I knew my career path was to be in direct clinical care. I became more and more interested in the emerging field of integrative medicine – an approach to healing that focuses on the whole person (body, mind and spirit), including all aspects of lifestyle. It emphasises the therapeutic relationship of person and practitioner and makes use of all scientifically supported therapies, both conventional, complementary and alternative.

I studied with Dolores Krieger, a retired nursing professor from NYU, every summer for ten years. She and Dora Kunz, a leader in the Theosophical Society of America, developed Therapeutic Touch, an energy healing technique based on the ancient practice of the 'laying on of hands'. This modality is used for the relief of pain and anxiety, and to ease the dying process. These two women mentored me in this healing practice, which opened me up to what I now understand as my spirituality – a lifelong quest to find meaning, purpose and comfort in the universality of human experience. Without the fear of being engulfed by my own feelings, they taught me how to connect deeply to a person. They helped me to trust the inherent capacity each human has to take responsibility for their healing and happiness.

In 1993 I was inspired by a television series produced by Bill Moyers entitled *Healing and the Mind*. The sixth episode described a weeklong retreat for people with cancer in Bolinas, California, run by Michael Lerner and Rachel Naomi Remen. I phoned Commonweal the following day and asked how I could learn more about their retreats. They happened to be offering their first workshop two months later to teach healthcare professionals how to run a cancer retreat programme and I registered.

After the Commonweal workshop, I gathered together a team of healthcare professionals who were interested in running cancer retreats, and the following year the Callanish Society was born in Vancouver. As I write this preface, Callanish has run almost one hundred weeklong retreats and has become a thriving centre for families with cancer to heal and strengthen into life, and for some, into death. It is a place dedicated to people who have been irrevocably changed by cancer, offering them retreats and programmes to reconnect to the essentials of life. We are committed to helping people talk about dying with those in their close relationships, to resolve past hurts and traumas, and to prepare themselves to die with peace and acceptance.

I hope *Radical Acts of Love* will give readers an increased understanding of the processes of dying, whether it be around one's own death, or the death of a loved one. Just as we carefully prepare for a birth, so too can we openly and consciously make preparations for dying, and therein provide some comfort and reassurance about what is, after all, a certainty for all of us. My wish is for this book to inspire hope for families who want to live and love as best they can in the period of time between learning of a poor prognosis and the moment of death itself.

The families in this book represent a small sector of the population and hence their experiences cannot be described in any way as universal. I am cognisant that some readers may not find their own experiences with death and dying represented in these stories and for that I am regretful.

I have tried to protect the privacy of the people in these stories by changing identifying features, or writing composite stories. I have sent stories to surviving family members to read for accuracy and comment. These communications have been deeply touching and have reassured me that love most certainly abides.

I have organised the book into four sections. Each one contains four to seven stories which will illuminate the experience of opening up to death, preparing for it, healing the past, dealing with unfinished business or accepting what is unresolved, making choices about dying on one's own terms, and learning to draw comfort from nature and the universality of death.

My Cree friend Maureen Kennedy told me that in her tradition, elders collect 'teaching stories' from their many years of life experiences.

'There comes a time,' she said, 'when the elders must release those stories into the world. You will know, Janie, when that time comes for you. You have many teaching stories by now, don't you?'

'Thirty years' worth, at least,' I said, nodding my head.

I believe the time for releasing these stories is now.

Preparing for death is a radical act of love for ourselves, and for those close to us who live on after we're gone. My hope is that these stories will reassure you, the reader, by providing a roadmap through one of the most important and least discussed experiences of our lives. May these teaching stories, gifted to me by others, heal, nourish and strengthen your hearts and reveal the terrible beauty inherent in living and dying that is your birthright.

I.

OPENING THE HEART TO DYING

'Peace comes when our hearts are open like the sky, vast as the ocean.'

—JACK KORNFIELD

At a retreat I attended a few years ago, Zoketsu Norman Fischer, a Soto Zen priest, offered a teaching that has stayed with me. He described how at the end of our life, when the body loses its functions, the heart continues to have an endless capacity to express and receive love. His statement comforts me, to know that even without a healthy body, we still have a worthy function: to give and receive love, opening our hearts in our living and dying so that our beloveds can be sustained by that love, long after we are gone.

I have learned that it is easier to open my heart in the presence of other people, than to do it on my own. Perhaps being open-hearted about any aspect of our life is dependent on our connection with other people. Maybe it is that very connection, especially

3

in difficult times, that activates our compassion and care towards one another and keeps us from feeling isolated and lonely.

I meet people every day who open their hearts to death, their own or another's; they show us how to remain open to the heartbreaks of life. They encourage us not to close up to pain and loss but to risk opening up to connection.

Opening the Heart to Dying contains five stories about what can happen to your life, and to the lives of those you love, when you open up to your own dying. Each of the five people in these stories made choices about dying that were congruent with the ways they had approached living. By opening their hearts to death, each person became more deeply connected and loving towards themselves and the people they cared about, and consequently more present in life itself.

I

KAREN: Golden Love

'Karen might be dying,' Kathy said on the phone one evening in early December, out of the blue.

'What do you mean?' I said, a wave of nausea rising from my gut. The three of us had been friends for twenty-five years. Eight years after we met, we co-founded the Callanish Society, a charity offering weeklong retreats for people living with cancer.

Kathy's voice was trembling. 'This past two weeks we both thought she had the flu, but every day she's weaker and she hasn't been off the couch for two days.'

My take-charge nursing voice kicked in. 'Has she seen a doctor?'

'You know what she's like, Janie. She'd rather not see a doctor,' Kathy said.

This was one of the sticking points in their twenty-three-year common-law relationship. Kathy was a nutritionist and preferred herbal potions over pharmaceuticals, like Karen, but they disagreed about the role of Western medicine in health and healing. Karen told me once how scared she was of doctors and hospitals because her father had died in a cancer hospital, after just one dose of chemotherapy, when she was in her twenties. She told me she believed it was the medicine, and not the cancer, that killed him.

'Kathy, you need to take her to the hospital,' I said.

The following morning, Kathy bundled Karen up in blankets and drove the eight miles to their doctor's office in town. They loved living in the Cariboo region of British Columbia, six hours north of Vancouver, with its big, snowy winters, swathes of grassland dotted with green lakes, and a multitude of wildlife. Kathy and Karen met in the Cariboo in their early twenties, when they both attended a conference held by the Emissaries of Divine Light, an intentional community with seven spiritual centres around the world. Several years after Karen and Kathy moved to live in the Emissary commune in the town of 100 Mile House, British Columbia, they fell in love.

The visit to the hospital confirmed Karen's liver

was failing. An ultrasound revealed widespread metastases from breast cancer. We knew what that meant: she likely wouldn't last long. We had worked with people with cancer for eighteen years by then and knew there was no rhyme nor reason for who gets it, what type or stage they are diagnosed with, who lives or dies from it, and how the dying process unfolds for each person. We knew that being a healthcare professional is no guarantee of good health, or an easy death.

By choosing not to consult an oncologist, Karen opted out of having any cancer treatment. She had always been clear and fast in her decision-making, not labouring over questions she already knew the answers to. She said it was all the fire in her astrology chart.

She was one of the few people I'd known to reject treatment without first learning the options. Many people find the reality of 'no treatment' too scary, and would rather adopt a fighting stance, with chemotherapy or radiation being their best weapons. Battling to stay alive made no sense to Karen. She knew her days were numbered and believed that even if treatment lengthened her life by some months, it wouldn't add to its quality. She had seen hundreds of people go through cancer treatment and felt that treatment in her case would just prolong the inevitable and zap what little physical energy she had. She wanted to feel as well as she could for as long as she could.

Karen chose to die at home with the support of her friends, family, and a local home care team, rather than die in a hospital or hospice. I knew where I needed and wanted to be. On 27 December 2013, I packed my bags for an indefinite amount of time and drove north to support my beloved friends as they conjured up the strength they would need for Karen's parting.

People have cared for dying loved ones at home for centuries, all around the world. Sometimes people need to be in hospital, because it's too hard to manage symptoms at home, but Karen was settled enough, and Kathy and I could administer the pain medications prescribed by her doctor. The home care nurse would also check in every day. I'd stay for as long as necessary to see Karen out of this world and be there to support Kathy.

'Will it be long?' Karen asked me, two days after I arrived. We were sitting at the kitchen table, over what ended up being our last bowl of soup together.

'Probably a week or so, at the most,' I replied. Sometimes there are surprises and people die quicker or slower than one predicts, but when you've seen many people die, your hunches are usually fairly accurate.

'That's good. I'm feeling okay about dying. Made it to sixty-two. Not bad,' she said. Karen had always treated life as an adventure and dying seemed to be no exception.

'I'm more scared of being kept alive than of dying,' she said, gazing out of the window for a few moments. 'Anyway, the place I'm going to *has* to supersede this existence on the earthly plane. I'm not scared. I'm just sad to die, to miss out on being on this beautiful earth with the people I love,' she said, looking at me. I felt a tear run down my cheek. Missing her had already begun to press into me.

'I hope you will at least come back, in some form, to tell us if you were right, that it *is* better over there,' I said.

'I imagine you passing your hand through the veil, like this,' she said, reaching for my hand across the table. 'I'll find you.'

'Wouldn't that be something if we really will be this close?' I said. 'Don't you wish we knew for sure?'

On the morning of 4 January, Karen told us to sing for her. 'Come on, you two minstrels. Get the ukuleles out.' Her voice was weak but the look in her blue eyes was as playful as ever. Over the years, whenever I became too serious she tried to make me lighten up. She never let me get too entrenched in an opinion, teasing me that my attachments to theories had little substance. Life was more of a mystery than a mental construct.

Kathy and I had taken up the ukulele six months before. We liked the idea of playing music, not just listening to it, and we thought it would help us relax during the tough times at work. Our ukulele teacher had assured us that with just three chords we could play two hundred songs. So far we'd managed five.

'Swing low, sweet chariot,' we sang, fumbling with the chords. 'Coming for to carry me home.'

Karen's eyes were closed, the inkling of a smile stretched across her chapped lips. She didn't have the strength to sing along.

'A band of angels coming after me, coming for to carry me home,' we crooned.

I could hardly believe how small Karen had become. She had always been such a fit, muscular woman, an avid tennis player until her late fifties. She joked about having a left bicep as large as Navratilova's. The weight had fallen off fast since her diagnosis in December, and her arms barely had the strength to lift a glass of water to her mouth.

The desire to eat and drink ceases at a certain point when the body no longer wants sustenance – a sign that death is near – but even with such a tiny body, Karen's presence in the room was enormous; mesmerising, like a harvest moon on a clear night.

'I looked over Jordan and what did I see,' Kathy and I strummed on. 'Coming for to carry me home.'

Karen was asleep, her head lolled to one side and her breath raspy. She slept for a couple of hours after that, and then awoke. Her half-opened eyes darted around the room as though she was tracking something compelling.

'I can only describe the place I go to when I'm half-awake with two words,' she told us: 'Golden love.'

'Golden love,' she repeated, and I felt a rush of reassurance relax my body. Kathy looked at me and smiled. There had been many shared moments of friendship when Karen's wisdom had disarmed us, dissolving any point of view we had thought worth holding on to.

'For years we've wondered what happens when we die? I have news for you,' she murmured. 'It *is* like we thought, but more, so much more. The great love that we come from is the same love that catches us at the end. It's so beautiful.'

Karen's words were like fragments of truth landing clickety-click into exactly the right place, the only possible configuration. She had always said spirit is the ubiquitous substance out of which each life arises

and passes away; she called this substance consciousness and said it was benevolent and eternal, like love.
Some people might name this loving substance God.
She didn't. She believed that when the body dies, the
energy that animated the physical form merges with
consciousness.

I have often wondered whether believing in the
continuity of the spirit helps us to feel more at peace
about dying. When dying is purely hypothetical, a
concept in the mind, believing in an afterlife often
reassures people. In my view, when the body *is* dying,
the visceral experience can be frightening, painful
and intolerable, or peaceful, comfortable and
manageable. Beliefs about the afterlife aren't what
make the difference between a difficult or an easeful
death, more the degree to which the body's symptoms
can be effectively managed, and the more a person
has made peace with the emotional experiences of his
or her life.

Karen had been unconscious for a couple of hours
when I sensed another change. Her breath was shal-
lower and the breaks between breaths lasted several
seconds. Her hands and feet were cool and mottled
and her lips pale. Death had been lingering in the
house for days, but had now moved closer.

'What's happening?' Kathy asked, feeling the shift
too.

'We'll stay right here with her,' I replied. Karen's eyelids fluttered, as if dreaming.

'Should we say goodbye?' Kathy asked.

'Do you want some time alone with Karen?'

'No, I just wondered if I should give her permission to go, tell her I'll be okay.' Kathy's face crumpled at the pain of imminent separation.

I moved from the foot of the bed to the head, where Kathy sat, and put my arm around her shoulder.

'We've been saying goodbye to Karen ever since we knew she was going to die,' I said, stroking Kathy's tousled hair. She hadn't slept much, lying on a mattress on the floor by Karen's bed the last two nights.

There's not one moment to say goodbye, but a series of moments through which the ending slowly unfolds.

Kathy leaned her body sideways onto the bed, her head resting on Karen's chest. 'I don't want to say goodbye. We've had such an amazing life together.'

Karen's breath was like a whisper, the out-breath slightly more audible than the in-breath.

'I can't imagine Karen needs permission to go, do you?' I said. 'She always was the boss.'

At this we both laughed, surrendering our attempts to move the situation along.

A dog barked a few houses away. The room was

quiet except for every so often when one of us said, 'I love you.' No other words made any sense.

Then the screen door banged against the side of the house and a rush of cold air pushed in on us. The wind had prised open the latch. We had opened the glass door earlier that afternoon so that Karen could feel the fresh air on her skin.

Tears flooded our eyes as we understood that the end was near. Ten seconds of stillness between breaths felt like forever. Another long exhalation, followed by silence – twenty seconds, thirty seconds. I knew to wait. Even after a minute there might be a final breath. And there it was. Karen breathed one more breath in and out, and then her life was over.

I didn't want to move a muscle, as though the still-ness in the room told me to wait, not to interfere with a cycle that was still completing in the room. My eyes were magnetised to the stand of poplars outside the window as they responded to a crescendo of wind and the sky that was turning deep pink as the sun dipped below the horizon. Then I noticed Karen's face was softening in tiny increments, the frown line between her eyebrows slowly dissolving and the shape of her mouth shifting. My attention was pulled back and forth between these two happenings: to the elemental world outside the window and to Karen's body, made up of elements too, which were shifting and dissolving in front of our eyes, in what seemed like a necessary dynamic interplay. About an hour later, the momentum in the room had ceased and I noticed a tiny smile had appeared on one side of Karen's mouth, as if to say, 'Yup, it's just as I thought.'

2

DANIEL: Memory Box

Daniel stood in the doorway of my counselling room, hand-in-hand with his seven-year-old daughter, Emily.

'Sorry for the surprise, Janie,' he said, glancing towards his daughter. 'Can Em entertain herself in the waiting room while I talk to you?' He looked at me from inside dark circles of fatigue. 'Lin came down with a migraine and stayed in bed this morning, and when Emily insisted on coming with me, I didn't have the heart to say no.'

Preventing the little disappointments was something he could do. He had no control over the big loss that lay ahead for her.

'My girls don't know how sick I am,' Daniel had told me on the phone the week before. 'It's better that way, don't you think?'

He'd decided not to tell them the latest news from the doctor, that his cancer had come back with a vengeance and he likely had only a few more months to live. Being the father of two daughters aged seven and nine was Daniel's proudest accomplishment.

'We need to have a longer chat about this in person, don't you think? Can you come in for a session?' I had asked.

Two days later he knocked on my door, Emily in tow.

She looked me straight in the eye, with a big smile. She exuded self-confidence, a sign of resilience, a character trait that makes all the difference in the aftermath of a tragedy.

'I'm so happy to finally meet you, Emily. I've heard lots about you.' I stooped down to her height and held out my hand. She took it briefly.

Emily's dark brown hair was cut into a bob with a fringe that fell shy of her wide hazel eyes. She was dressed in multiple shades of pink. Her sneakers were well-worn and the strobe lights in the heels flickered faintly as she headed for one of the comfy chairs. She pulled a colouring book and a zip-lock bag of crayons out of her backpack.

'If you need us, just knock on this door, okay?' I pointed to the door of my counselling room. 'Your daddy and I will be in there talking.'

She nodded without looking up. She was already colouring the dress of Princess Aurora bright purple.

Daniel took his usual seat on the overstuffed couch with its back to the window. His baldness seemed to highlight the ashen complexion of a man losing his life force, and his baggy sweatsuit attempted to obscure his weight loss.

A large maple tree against a backdrop of blue sky filled my office window behind where Daniel sat. The tree steadied me for conversations that were not often easy.

'My wife and her parents are relying on me to get better. When I talk about dying, they tell me to stop being so negative. They don't want to talk about death and believe that talking about it will make it happen. There are beliefs in her culture which I don't understand. Of course I want to live, but it's not a reality any more, is it?' Daniel held my gaze and I inhaled slowly.

In these moments, when someone directly asks if they are dying, there are choices to make in response. Slip beneath the words, shift my eyes away from the gaze, succumb to the instinct to protect, to avoid the pain, to say something else, anything else. *You can beat this cancer. You're too young to die. Miracles happen, they really do. I know lots of people who've defied their prognoses. Michael, the guy you met last time you were here, outlived the doctor's prediction by two years.* You want to echo a family's plea that death is conquerable, that the sick person just has to find the strength to fight. But in the end, you have to be honest. Death was already present on the couch beside Daniel, coaxing me to speak, and Daniel needed me to respect his capacity to handle the truth. Without respect, there's no dignity.

I exhaled slowly. 'No, it's not looking like you're going to make it, Daniel.'

Daniel's voice was urgent. 'If I'm going to die, then I want it to be as easy as possible for Lin and the kids. They've got to be able to manage without me.' He turned his wedding band around and around on his finger, loose from the weight loss.

'Daniel, I can help you prepare for your death, without either of us giving up hope that surprising things can happen.' Daniel's shoulders dropped an inch or two as he relaxed, and his eyes gave way to tears of relief.

'Thank God. I knew I couldn't figure this out by myself. I just know that pretending I'm *not* going to die isn't going to help anyone,' he said.

The dawning reality that death cannot be avoided has its own rhythm, its own season, and fruitful conversations about dying happen in their right time. I used to think it was my duty as a healthcare professional to guide people towards the fact that death was approaching, even without an invitation into the conversation. I'd feel a sudden rush of heat in my body, an upwelling of responsibility. I believed my forthrightness would help the dying person and give them enough time to prepare for what was ahead. I had seen many people run out of time to say goodbye, which often precipitates years of regret for those left behind.

However, over time, I've learned that my agenda, my hurry to open up a conversation, can frighten a person who isn't ready. I've had to cultivate patience, quell the impulse to jump in until the truth has caught up and the psyche has assimilated what the body already knows. Sometimes the mind never catches up, and I have had to learn to accept that, too.

I knew Daniel was ready to talk from the urgency in his voice and the way he leaned forward into our conversation.

'Let's start with the practical stuff,' I said, an easier place to start than the emotional preparation. 'Have you thought about where you might die?' I asked.

'I can't imagine Lin and the kids coping if I die at home, in our bed. She'd be haunted after. What do you think?' he asked.

'Memories of death are not always gruesome. They can be gentle and afterwards people usually speak about the comfort of having the person die at home,' I said.

Daniel's face was softer. 'My grandpa died in his own bed, now that I think of it, and Grandma seemed to be okay, but Lin believes death is unlucky so I think it would be easier for her if I died in a hospital, or a hospice,' Daniel said.

I explained to Daniel the difference between palliative care units, regular medical units and hospices. Palliative care units (PCUs) and hospices tend to be better staffed than medical units, and have team members who are specialised in end-of-life care. They both have less of an institutional atmosphere. People tend to go to a PCU for symptom management, such as pain or nausea, and then, once that's under control, they can go home again or to a hospice. Most hospices have a policy of only admitting people who have a prognosis of three to six months.

A faint flush of pink had settled in Daniel's cheeks. The knowledge that help was tangible likely brought him some ease and consolation.

'There's a hospice quite near your house. You can bring things from home such as pictures for the walls and your own pillows and bedding. Lin and the kids could be there as much as they want, and they can even sleep over,' I said. Daniel's eyes were locked onto mine.

Memories of countless families I had known flooded my mind. Little Sarah, who was four when her mom died in a hospice, brought offerings from home: a flower from the garden, a candy, a storybook. The hurt was evident in her wary glances and the dishevelled state of her mismatched clothes. Matthew, almost sixteen, who slumped in the chair by the window of his dad's hospital room, baseball cap pulled down low, earbuds always in place. He exuded inaccessibility, but he never missed a day of the fifteen-day after-school vigil before his dad died.

Daniel moved himself from the practical to the emotional. 'Is it okay for the kids to see me dying? Would it traumatise them?'

'It depends on whether the process is an easeful one or not. Most times the palliative care team can settle your symptoms, and you'd look to the kids like you were sleeping. It will be very sad for them, but not traumatic.' I was aware of my change in emphasis, from 'would' to 'will', ushering Daniel closer to what was inevitable. He leaned forward slowly to pick up the glass of water on the table and took a couple of gulps. I waited while he took a tissue and wiped his mouth, then dropped the tissue into the wastepaper basket. When he lifted his eyes to mine, I continued.

'In the unusual circumstance there is a symptom that's difficult to control, or something sudden happens, then it is best for kids not to be there. That *would* be traumatic,' I said.

'Who decides?' Daniel asked, with surprising stamina for what had become a lengthy conversation. My thoughts briefly turned to Emily in the waiting room. I felt grateful for her self-reliance that allowed me to talk to her dad without interruption.

'The team at the hospice will guide you, but it would be good to talk with Lin about this too.'

'What about after I've died? Can the kids see me then?' Daniel asked.

I reassured Daniel that children usually know whether or not they want to see the person who has died, and how long they want to stay in the room. I recommended that his wife Lin or someone close to the kids should be with them. Kids need to say goodbye just as much as adults do.

'This might sound like a weird question.' Daniel paused, then looked at me.

'It's okay,' I said.

'How am I going to know when I'm dying? Are you living one day, and dying the next?'

'We live right up until the last breath, really, but there is a time when we enter the final phase of dying which usually lasts from a few hours to a few days. The body doesn't want food or liquids any more, and the organs naturally shut down. You'll be asleep more than awake, and you will likely know you are dying,' I said.

Daniel leaned back against the cushions of the couch and glanced behind him, out of the window, taking a break from the conversation.

He turned back and I continued. 'When Lin entered the last phase of childbirth, the pushing part, you were there, right? No matter how much determination she had, she couldn't stop what was happening. Your daughters really birthed themselves,' I said.

Daniel's eyes shone at the memory. 'It was amazing to hold each of them for the first time.'

When I told him my belief that just as the body knows how to birth itself, it also knows how to die, I saw the relief soften his face.

'Death will happen when it happens,' he nodded.

I waited to see if there was more, or whether Daniel would close the conversation. He might have used up all his extra energy for the day, and he still had to drive home.

His voice had become subdued. 'I just hate all the pressure to have to will this cancer away with my mind. The stress comes from all those books Lin keeps leaving by my bed, the ones that tell me that my mind is stronger than the cancer. If I could do that, I would have already done it, right? Of course I want to live, but this cancer has got the better of me.' He paused, as though an unbidden thought was pushing up against him. 'This is not my fault is it, Janie, getting cancer?'

24

'Of course it's not your fault,' I said, with a vehemence that surprised me. 'Life deals us this stuff and then we have to handle it, and how we do that affects not just our own life but the lives of all the people we love, into the next generation and the next. If you can find compassion for yourself, Daniel, then your daughters will learn from you. Your dignity and self-respect will accompany them throughout their lives.' I felt the warmth of emotion build up behind my eyes at the thought of his daughters growing up without this fine man.

Daniel had perked up, sitting taller, as though his hope was being redefined. Instead of hoping for survival, he could hope for continued meaningful moments with his family, for as long as possible.

'Perhaps we should check on Emily?' Daniel suggested. I stood up and opened the door to the waiting room. Emily looked up expectantly.

She entered the counselling room and plonked herself down on the couch close to her dad and looked at me with wide eyes.

'What were you and Daddy talking about?' she asked.

I looked at Daniel to determine if he wanted to speak. He nodded at me to respond.

'Your daddy and I were talking about what it's like to be sick.'

Emily looked up at her dad. His eyes were moist.

'Do you know what's going on with your daddy?' I asked.

'Yes, he has cancer, and he's going to die,' Emily said, matter-of-factly.

I raised my eyes to the maple outside, to seek brief solace from the heartbreak of the moment, and I noticed the new tender leaves shivering in the April breeze. When I looked at Daniel, a plea for help radiated from his eyes.

I took his cue and responded. 'It will be very sad for you and your mommy, and for your sister, won't it, when Daddy dies?' I said. Choosing to be honest in a situation like this feels like jumping into an abyss.

'Yes, it will,' she said. 'Daddy, I don't want you to die.'

She looked up at him and Daniel reached out with both arms and drew her in against his frail body. Witnessing the intimacy of father and daughter took me to my own father dying, and to all the daughters and sons who must say goodbye to parents too soon. I felt oddly comforted by remembering my father's love and the deep ache of my own loss.

Daniel whispered into Emily's ear. 'I'll always love you, Em, no matter whether I'm here or not. Will you remember that?' Her head acknowledged his question with a slight nod. Daniel continued, 'I would move a mountain or drink the whole ocean or never eat another candy if it meant I could stay here and be your dad.'

'Would you eat Muffy's cat food?' Emily looked up with a mischievous smile.

'I most certainly would,' he said.

Emily smacked her lips together in satisfaction. 'Good.'

I leaned towards her. 'Sometimes it can help to talk about the things you're going to miss when Daddy dies, because they become the happy memories that can help you feel better when you're sad,' I said.

Emily's eyes lit up. 'I'd like to talk about those things.'

'Maybe you and Daddy can make a memory box together? First, you remember all the things you love about Daddy, and then you find something at home or make something to put in the box to remind you of that special memory. We could start talking about the memories today, and then when you go home, perhaps you and Claire can finish the memory box together, with your dad?'

Emily nodded with enthusiasm.

'What is one thing you love about Daddy?' I asked.

Without any hesitation she answered, 'I love Daddy's kisses.' She smiled up at him.

'Of course you do,' I said. 'How do you think we

could put Daddy's kisses in the memory box, so that you can pull one out when you want to remember?'

'I know,' she said, excitedly. 'I could put Mommy's lipstick on Daddy and then he could kiss pieces of paper and then we could put them in the box.' She giggled.

Daniel and I looked at one another with raised eyebrows. Creativity had wrapped the pain of imminent loss in delight. His kisses would survive long after he was gone.

'Daddy, what do you think? Will you do it?' Emily asked.

'Of course,' Daniel said.

We talked then about other ideas for objects to go in the memory box. Children sometimes choose favourite photographs from vacations or celebrations, or saved letters or cards written from one to the other. Some parents write letters to their children or make audiotapes or videos of them reading favourite stories. Children might pick items of clothing, or jewellery, or objects from nature like shells or rocks collected from a special beach. They might paint and decorate the memory box together.

'Will you bring your memory box to show me next time you come?' I asked Emily. She nodded.

Children need to make preparations, too.

* * *

Lin asked her daughters if they wanted to see their dad after he died and they both said they did. Daniel had been admitted to hospital suddenly one day when his pain had escalated and he died forty-eight hours later, from what the doctor thought was likely a blood clot. Lin thought the girls might want to do something special for their dad, and she left it up to them to decide what they wanted that to be.

Emily asked Lin if she and her sister Claire could take all the petals off the flowers in the vases along the window ledge, and she had agreed. The girls then slowly and carefully pulled the petals off each flower and piled them up on the tray table next to the bed. There were tulips and lilies, anemones and roses, petals of all sizes and colours, and some that still held fragrance. The girls carefully overlapped the petals, one at a time, and shaped them into the words 'WE LOVE YOU DADDY' on top of the white blanket covering Daniel's lifeless body. All the while they did this, they chatted to him, telling him the stories they would never forget.

3

RACHEL: Pod of Orcas

Rachel asked me to check the small lump on her inner right thigh, just above her knee.

'It feels like a cyst,' I said, my fingers palpating the interloper just under the surface of Rachel's skin. I didn't think for a moment it could be cancer. Malignancies are usually fixed and hard to the touch.

Rachel had been a bedside nurse, like me, for many years before she became a nurse educator and I became a clinical nurse specialist. Every summer for ten years we registered for the same Therapeutic Touch workshop, on Orcas Island, to enhance our skills and catch up on each other's lives. Rachel and I always looked forward to it.

My phone rang a couple of weeks later.

'Brace yourself,' Rachel said. The pause felt

interminable. I could hear her rapid breaths. 'The lump you felt on my leg is a sarcoma. My oncologist told me he might have to amputate my leg.' Her voice cracked.

'Oh, shit. I'm so sorry, Rachel,' I said. I knew not all sarcomas required such radical surgery, but I also knew that if surgical amputation was given as an option with such an aggressive cancer, they were going for a cure. This diagnosis would mean several hours of surgery followed by multiple rounds of chemotherapy and months of rehabilitation. Just three weeks after celebrating her sixtieth birthday, Rachel would have to find more fortitude than anyone should have to. She had already gone through breast cancer ten years earlier, but this was a new primary cancer, a different beast altogether.

'Sarcoma is not good, is it?' she asked.

I inhaled deeply but didn't want to pause for too long before I answered. 'It depends on the pathology, doesn't it? Let's not get too far ahead until we have more information,' I said, trying to suppress the fear swirling in the pit of my stomach. The cancer was one nightmare, the amputation another.

Rachel didn't need me to say, 'Hey, you're a fighter. You've been through cancer before and beaten it. You can do it again.'

People become disoriented and vulnerable when

the fear of death snatches ordinary life out from under them, the moment destiny reveals itself. It's not the time for bravado from friends.

Grappling for words that were slow in coming, I tried to push my love down the phone line, hoping she'd feel it.

'I wish I was with you right now. You'll get through this, one step at a time.'

I heard the whimper of her crying and felt the urge to move the conversation along. Had Rachel been in the chair across from me I'd have held her hand, my love more easily conveyed through physical touch.

'What happens next?' I asked.

'I'm coming to town next week to see the surgeon, Dr Lestin. Have you heard of him?' she asked.

'The word on the street says that he's the best, though he doesn't get such high marks for bedside manner,' I said.

'If I had to choose one quality over another, I'd rather he be good with his hands than be a good listener, wouldn't you?' she replied. 'I can get my emotional support from other people.'

'I suppose,' I said, wishing he could be one of those doctors who was an expert on both counts. The doctors I know who are brilliant surgeons and excellent communicators understand it is the emotional relationship, as well as the expertise, that builds resilience in people to tackle what would feel impossible without both. We rise up to meet an experience when we know someone cares about us.

'Could you come to the appointment? Another set of ears would help. Michael and I will be pretty stressed out,' she said.

'Of course.' I knew she'd be there for me if I were in the same spot.

A few days later, on a rainy November day, Rachel and her husband caught an early ferry to Vancouver. They were sitting side by side on beige plastic waiting-room chairs at the hospital when I tracked them down. The room was packed, though nobody conversed; an eerie quiet that exuded uncertainty. Michael held an unopened newspaper on his lap and rested one arm loosely across Rachel's shoulders. His forehead wrinkled as he gazed at the wall of patient-education brochures across the room. Rachel looked surprisingly cheerful. She wore a long indigo cardigan over black jeans and her deep blue eyes intensified the white of her thick, straight, shoulder-length hair.

'Hey there, Janie. Sorry to get you out of bed so early,' Rachel said brightly, as she stood up to greet me.

'Couldn't think of anywhere else I'd rather be,'

I said with a grin. I hugged her, then Michael, and sat down on the only vacant chair.

Forty minutes after the scheduled appointment time, a nurse called loudly from the nurses' station, 'Rachel McLeod. In there.' She pointed to a door and walked away.

The doctor's office looked like a physiotherapist's room, with coloured gym balls of different sizes pushed into one corner and a collection of weights stacked neatly along a rack in another. Wheelchairs, walkers, crutches and canes were set along one wall, and a treadmill with sturdy handrails sat in the middle of the room.

Dr Lestin slid off the table on which he had been sitting when we entered. A thin paper chart lay on the table. 'RACHEL MCLEOD' was written in red ink along one edge of the file folder that contained her future. He shook Rachel's hand, then Michael's, and nodded at me briefly. He gestured for us to sit down.

'Let's cut to the chase, shall we? We both know why you're here.' Without waiting for a response, the doctor continued. 'I'm afraid we have a very serious situation here that requires immediate and extensive surgery.' He looked down at his shiny brogues, perhaps hoping they would walk him away. Direct eye contact might have helped to soften the blow.

'Say more,' Rachel encouraged, as though she was talking about someone else.

'Well, I always hope to salvage the leg, but in your case I can't. We need to take off the leg and fit you with a prosthesis. Most people do very well, and with good physiotherapy you'll be back on your feet, so to speak, within a couple of months.'

He smiled as his quip fluttered in the air and landed heavily on the grey linoleum beneath our feet. *The* leg, rather than *your* leg, suggested it had to be difficult to deliver such information.

'Oh, and the good news: this cancer hasn't spread anywhere else in your body,' he said.

Rachel jumped out of the chair and with a smile said, 'So now I know why I've practised yoga all these years. The tree pose, one of my favourites.'

She tucked the sole of her right foot high up on her left inner thigh, balancing steadily on her left leg. She raised both arms up over her head with her palms pressed together. She showed how flexible she was and how adaptable she would be with only one leg. Rachel had always had a quirky sense of humour, and I could see that Dr Lestin was not sure whether to smile.

He had other patients to see, made evident by the speed of his words and his backing up towards the door. 'Okay, I want to get you in sometime in the next week or two. The anaesthetist will see you the morning of surgery. Any questions?'

Rachel looked at Michael, who shook his head. No questions. Shock can seize the mind in these kinds of interactions between doctor and patient, and freeze any questions until later, when they arise, often in the quiet of night. Doctors sometimes give patients only one opportunity for questions after delivering bad news, and time feels pressured. A question Rachel might have asked if she had had time to assimilate the information would have been: *Could I have a moment, please?* Or, *When questions do come up later, how can I reach you?*

Grasping the doctor's outstretched hand as we headed towards the door, I surprised myself by saying, 'Thank you. This isn't an easy path you've chosen. Very few could do your job. I appreciate you being there for my friend.'

His composure softened, and as our eyes met I felt the impact of hundreds, if not thousands, of past patients' reactions and rejections, people who were so shocked by bad news that they'd attempted to shoot the messenger. I hoped that Rachel had noticed the shift in his expression.

The attempt to humanise healthcare professionals comes naturally to me now, after years of witnessing professional–patient interactions lacking warmth and connection. We are educated to create distance between ourselves and our patients, supposedly to protect us from the difficult emotions that inevitably arise within us. I believe this distance actually de-humanises the professional and the patient, and it removes the possibility for an authentic and mutually caring relationship. I believe this caring relationship often provides the foundation for a sound recovery.

Dr Lestin reached for Rachel's hand and quickly shook it, while his eyes landed on the file folder in his left hand. 'See you soon then,' he said, as he opened the door to let himself out.

Sipping lattes in the coffee shop down the street from the hospital later that morning, I asked Rachel how she could be so calm in the meeting with her surgeon.

'I have a story to tell you,' she said.

She recounted how she'd dragged herself out of bed that morning with an enormous sense of dread at the prospect of meeting the doctor. He would tell her the results of the tests and whether the sarcoma had spread to other parts of her body. He would also recommend the type of surgery she was to undergo.

Rachel had slumped low in her seat on the ferry, oblivious to the presence of Michael, her husband of twenty-five years, beside her. She told me that she felt as though she was alone on a raft set adrift at sea, no way back to shore, and no land in sight. About fifteen minutes after departure, Rachel recalled being vaguely aware of hearing an announcement over the ferry's PA system. She heard Michael mutter some-thing about a pod of orcas off the starboard bow. Rachel shook her head when he suggested she come out on deck with him. She remembered looking down at her running shoes and noticing that her laces were undone. She hadn't bothered to tie them up when she'd left the house earlier that morning.

I don't want to go out in the rain. I've seen orcas before. I'll see them again, she thought. She felt unlike herself, estranged from the person who loved to kayak in the Johnstone Strait and sleep outside on warm summer nights.

Suddenly, a strong invisible tug pulled Rachel up and out of her seat, a force too powerful to resist. She stepped outside into the wild and blustery early morning light. The sea was steely grey and the almost-black sky merged with the ocean at the horizon. The ship's deck glistened in the wet and the rain pelted her uncovered head, plastering her hair to her scalp as the wind pushed open her unzipped fleece jacket. She noticed Michael and three other people huddled together at the furthest point forward on the starboard deck, looking out to sea.

Joining them, she leaned over the deck's railing and saw the first flash of black and white as a large orca surfaced about one hundred feet from the ferry. A thrill of delight coursed through her body. Soon she counted seven or eight orcas, surfacing and diving in and around one another, their dorsal fins pointing to the sky. A plume of spray from a blowhole shot up into the air before the orca disappeared beneath the surface of the frothy backwash. A couple of young ones mimicked their mothers, dipping and diving, and Rachel knew that this was likely a resident pod, which would include up to four generations.

Standing on the deck in the wind and rain that day, Rachel thought it was likely just a lucky moment, seeing the orcas, but she hoped it was more than that. She wanted to believe they had come to support her, to lift her out of her isolation and despair. She had read that when one orca in a pod gets sick, the others take turns supporting their ailing family member from beneath.

Rachel's perspective expanded. She sensed a lineage of multiple generations of west-coast people who had lived and died along that shoreline for thousands of years. No matter how long she lived, she knew she'd always be remembered within that collective story. Whatever the surgeon would tell her later that morning, whether she would die soon or live for a long time, it didn't matter.

Life was unfolding for her, as it had for countless people and species throughout time. At that moment of expanded awareness Rachel had fallen into a profound stillness. She called it grace. She told me that the peacefulness had stayed with her all the way through the meeting with Dr Lestin.

Eight days later, I made my way through a series of *Staff Only* doors to the intensive care unit. Working in hospitals gave me the confidence to push through forbidden doors. Unconscious patients attached to ventilators, tubes and IVs occupied most of the beds. Diligent nurses with clipboards in their hands monitored screens and forgot about their lives at home. Every so often a machine alarm would beep, requiring attention.

I had promised Rachel I would do Therapeutic Touch as soon after her surgery as possible. We had both read the research that confirms that this energy work can significantly decrease pain after surgery, and especially phantom limb pain.

I leaned over and kissed Rachel on the cheek. The peppery smell of anaesthesia lingered on her breath and she looked like most post-op patients do the day after surgery, tired and relieved.

She smiled wanly. 'Thanks so much for coming. How are you?'

'I'm happy to see you,' I said. 'How's the pain?'

'Oh, I'm hooked up to this gizmo,' she said, pulling back the bedcovers. Rachel showed me the patient-controlled analgesia pump that was attached to fine tubing inserted into the epidural space, between two of her vertebrae. This method is the most effective way to control post-operative pain, and Rachel could give herself extra doses of medication when she needed it.

'Right now I'm doing great. Michael just stepped out for a bite to eat, so your timing is perfect. How about some Therapeutic Touch?' she asked.

'That's why I'm here.' I am always glad to offer something practical in a situation like this, when one can often feel helpless. Rachel and I had practised and taught Therapeutic Touch for years, and I had seen the technique relax countless people in pain within three to four minutes. I didn't have to fully understand how moving my hands slowly from head to toe, a few inches above a person's body, could have such a profoundly relaxing effect. 'Has Michael still not learned how to do TT?' I laughed at the standing joke between us. He was sceptical even though he had been a recipient of TT many times and always liked how relaxed he felt. The relaxation effect is independent of whether a person believes in the therapy or not.

Anxiety fluttered in my stomach as I gently pulled down the bedcovers. I calmed myself by closing my eyes for a few minutes. I silently wished Rachel and everyone in the intensive care unit a good recovery.

A familiar feeling of tranquillity washed through me as I placed my right hand under the sole of Rachel's only foot, and my left hand gently on her ankle. I heard her soft exhalation as she began to settle. I held her foot for two or three minutes and imagined any tension flowing out of the sole into my hands, and down my body through my feet and into the ground. I then tiptoed to the head of the bed and began to slowly move my hands downwards in broad strokes, a few inches above her body, from the top of her head, down her torso to her left leg and foot, including the empty space that her right leg and foot had once inhabited. According to Dolores Krieger, the founder of this technique, if the practitioner is calm and grounded, the patient will relax more quickly than if he or she is anxious. I find the process calms me.

I invoked the pod of orcas in my mind, and the ease with which they travel vast distances through space, and I wished that Rachel be graced with such ease as she learned a new way to move through her world. I watched the muscles of her face soften and her eyelids twitch as a dream passed through. Her breathing slowed and deepened as she drifted off to sleep.

Rachel and I no longer go to the summer workshops together on Orcas Island but we connect by phone or email from time to time. We both lead busy, active lives. Rachel's surgery was almost twenty years ago and her cancer has never returned.

4

JOHN: Fear Disappears

'Such a cliché, I know, but honestly, I can't believe this happened to me.'

John wrung his forty-eight-year-old hands.

'But really, why *not* me? I see enough of it in my family practice. Out of the blue. Cancer. But this is not a good cancer. You and I both know lung cancer is often a death sentence, don't we?' He pierced me with the question.

'I'm so sorry,' I said.

This was my first meeting with John. He had left a voicemail the week before. 'Can you fit me in for counselling? My oncologist said to call you.' He sounded in control then, as though he was making a referral for one of his patients. He had worked as a family doctor for over two decades.

'At least my kids are doing well, one at university,

and two almost there. I'm proud of them. They'll do okay.' His cheeks were wet. The Kleenex box was close. I leave a person to reach for a tissue rather than interrupt the flow of emotion to offer one.

When life meets death, some people strive to hold the edges of their lives together, carry on as best they can with work, with family life, with some semblance of normality. They allow their lives to dissolve slowly and only when necessary. John was different. He made a clean break.

I have noticed that some people handle transitions with relative ease and some with great difficulty: a person might return to work from vacation and slide back into the routine appreciative of their holiday adventures; or they might take several days to readjust to being back at work, reminiscing about their vacation and perseverating on whether they really like their job after all. A bereaved spouse may find ways to grieve and also invite in a new relationship a few months after the death, one experience not inhibiting the other. Other grieving people find life without their loved one unbearable and take many months or even years to be social again, and some never do. I imagined that John had likely been a person who navigated change with relative ease.

'Even if this chemo works for a while, it won't keep me alive for long. Last week I sent a letter to all my

45

patients and told them I have incurable cancer and that I'm leaving my practice. They're all terribly upset but it's what I have to do,' he said. 'I love my work but now it's about me, and my family.'

Early on in relationships with clients I search for core strengths. What kind of support and encouragement did they receive growing up? Did adults believe in them? Were they safe? Did they feel loved? If not, has their sense of self been strengthened or diminished by life's challenges?

John's strength of character was obvious: the way he held my gaze, the timbre of his voice, the uprightness of his spine, his ability to see beyond his own heartache.

John came to see me twice a month for counselling. During one session, six months after we first met, his demeanour had shifted and he seemed less sure of himself. His strength of character was diminished somehow, and I noticed the weight loss and shortness of breath.

'My fear is unstoppable. I'm scared all the time.' His eyes met mine. 'I think about dying constantly.'

Resilience doesn't guarantee fearlessness; nor does being a physician.

'It's intense to feel the grip of fear like that,' I said. 'As you know from your patients, a body is hardwired

RADICAL ACTS OF LOVE

for survival, and when under threat the flight-or-fight response pumps adrenaline and cortisol into the nervous system. The good news is that we can learn to tell the difference between a real and a perceived threat. You can learn to dissipate imaginary fear.'

'Great. Will you please take me out of my misery?' John smiled at the inkling of relief.

'Fear is like a fog that infiltrates everything. If we dissect our fears into specifics, to discover exactly what it is that frightens us, we become less of a victim to fear, and less controlled by it. Are you up for trying to identify your fears?' I asked.

'Can't think of anything I'd rather do,' he quipped. 'Sure, why not, if you think it'll help.' John's hand was shaking slightly as he took the writing pad I offered him. He pulled a fountain pen out of his top-left blazer pocket. 'I love this pen. It's the one I wrote my prescriptions with.'

As John inscribed, I noticed the large framed photograph on the wall to my left, a gift to myself from a trip to Arizona. The image of sunlight illuminating the sandstone walls of Antelope Canyon, narrowly carved into a slot over centuries by flash floods, comforted me. Seeing how beauty in nature can be created from unpredictable weather patterns reminded me of the people navigating their own extreme weather patterns, to emerge worn but somehow finer.

I knew John would need enough time to be thorough. Fears can hide in the darkest corners of a psyche. His list soon spilled onto a second page.

Fear is most often evoked by thoughts of the future or the past. One way to lessen fear's grip is through simple distraction into present time. An activity that takes one's attention from the inner world of thoughts and feelings into the tangible world of body and movement and engagement with another person can release the control fear has over us. As I watched John's hand move across the paper, I sensed that although his mind was focusing on fearful thoughts, the simple gesture of writing was transferring the thoughts from inside his mind out onto the page. The act of writing could well be helping to quell his fears.

John screwed the gold lid back onto his pen.

'Would you read your list aloud?' I asked.

'Okay.' John uncrossed his ankles and straightened his back, assuming a formal posture for reading. I imagined he had given many presentations during his professional life.

'*Fear of missing out.*

Fear of dying with regrets.

Fear of Natalie finding a new husband too soon.'

He paused and looked up from the page. 'This is harder than I thought.'

I nodded. 'Take your time, no rush.'

'*Fear of Natalie screwing up the finances and not leaving enough for the kids.*

Fear of Natalie not coping without me.

Fear of dying in pain.

Fear of suffocating.

Fear of dying in hospital with tubes and catheters.'

John rubbed the palm of his hand over his nose and mouth as though brushing away the intrusion of life support.

'*Fear of others having to deal with my work files.*

Fear of being too dependent on my family.

Fear of my mother having a nervous breakdown.

Fear of losing my sense of humour.

Fear of my dog dying before me.'

His voice dropped to a whisper for the losses that were barely utterable.

'*Fear of saying goodbye.*

Fear of not existing.

Fear of lingering on too long.

Fear of my fear.

Fear of dying alone.'

John let out a big sigh, took off his reading glasses and lifted his head.

'See why I can't sleep at night?'

'I do,' I said. 'What are you aware of, now you have spoken your fears aloud?'

'They feel smaller, like I'm in charge, like they

can't control me,' he said. 'And I'm aware of something else, too, that's harder to describe, a settling deep inside me that I'm going to be okay, no matter what happens.'

'You might have noticed there are some fears on your list that we can do something about, and others that are not so easy,' I said. 'Would you bring Natalie with you next time so we can talk about some of the fears that relate to her?'

'I'm not sure she's ready,' he said.

'Most people aren't ready to lose the ones they love,' I replied.

John blinked back tears. 'I'll ask her.'

Two weeks later Natalie and John arrived for a session. They sat side-by-side on the couch and John's right hand rested on her thigh. I noticed his fingernails were faintly blue, a sign that there was not enough oxygen circulating through his bloodstream.

Natalie's dark hair was swept back by a wide tortoise-shell clasp, revealing her large brown eyes and delicate features. Her lips bore a fresh coat of bright red lipstick. She clenched John's hand and tried not to cry.

'He's my soulmate,' she said. 'I knew it the moment we met back in the early nineties. Don't get me wrong, we fight like cat and dog sometimes. Did he tell you how stubborn he is?'

I shook my head. 'Somehow that doesn't surprise me, though.' I looked back and forth from one face to the other. 'I'm glad you found your soulmate. Makes this all so terribly sad, though, doesn't it?'

Natalie's face collapsed. 'I can't talk about this. I really can't.' Dabbing her cheeks quickly with a tissue, she then blew her nose hard. She glanced sideways at John.

'Okay, you talk and I'll listen. Maybe I can manage that,' she said.

John looked at me. I nodded.

'Nat, I've started to explore my fears here because, as you well know, even though I take a sedative every night to sleep, I wake up terrified every morning. Some of my fears are related to you.' He looked over at her.

'Go on,' she said.

His voice trembled and his eyes searched for mine.

I sent back a look that said, *Keep going*.

'This might sound weird, but I'm scared you'll move on too fast after I'm gone, find someone else. Maybe it'd be okay eventually, hon. I'd want that for you, but not too soon.' His voice was small.

'Are you serious?' Natalie asked. 'Do you think I'll have time? I'll be a single parent, don't forget.' Her black eyebrows cinched and then just as quickly relaxed.

Her voice softened. 'Besides, you're irreplaceable. Really, you are. And who else would put up with me?' She reached up with her left hand and stroked his hollowed cheek.

John spoke quietly into his chest as a regret bubbled to the surface.

'I haven't talked here about what I did all those years back, when I had the affair, and you forgave me, but I still haven't forgiven myself, you know? You took me back, but I hate what I did.'

'Oh, for goodness' sake. Are you still on about that? Take it to your grave if you want, but please let it go, for your own sake.' Natalie looked at me for help.

'It sounds like Natalie has forgiven you. What stops you from forgiving yourself?' I asked.

'I loathe myself for what I did to her. I don't know how to forgive myself. I sometimes think I deserve to die.'

My heart skipped a beat, as it does sometimes when a glimmer emerges from the deep. I've heard this kind of confession before. A person believing their cancer was a punishment for wrongdoing. Remorse is a helpful human emotion in that it evokes compassion for loved ones we have hurt, and we can take responsibility. Guilt is unhelpful in that it is based in self-loathing, which separates us from the people we love.

Natalie leaned into him. 'John, honey. You don't deserve to die. You're an amazing husband. You did one stupid thing, but you are human. Please move on.'

Then she broke down.

John placed his hand on top of hers and stroked gently from her wrist to her fingertips and back. 'I'm just sorry, sweetheart, for hurting you.' She looked up at him, her eyes soft with tenderness. 'And I'm so sorry I'm going to die. Sorry for me, for you, for all of us,' he said.

She nodded. 'Me too. I'm going to miss you terribly.' Natalie rested her head against John's bony shoulder and he wrapped all the energy he had left around her.

The space in the room amplified in the quiet. I heard the tick of the clock and the cars whoosh by in the rain outside.

Over the next two months, we explored each of John's fears. Sometimes it was John and me, and other sessions included Natalie, or John's mother. There were a few times when all three kids came, with or without their parents.

When John was too sick to come, I drove half an hour to their home. He got dressed when he could and we'd meet by the fire in the den, at one end of the big family kitchen. When he was too tired to come downstairs, he welcomed me into his large bright bedroom with a view onto the old dogwood tree. Natalie lay on the bed beside him for our talks and inevitably Shadow, their Border Collie, would curl up on the floor at my feet.

I asked John one afternoon, as the crocuses had just begun to pop their heads out of the cold ground: 'How's the fear?'

'You know, it's weird, but the fear has disappeared. All those fears I wrote about when we first identified the list three months ago don't plague me any more. Why is that?' John turned his head to look me in the eye. I noticed the whites of his eyes were a pale yellow, a sign his liver was failing.

'You've worked hard at dispelling your fears. You've faced your demons and that's liberating. Fear is left with nothing to hold on to when we accept how little control we have over our lives,' I said.

John continued. 'Dying isn't as scary as I thought. You just have to be willing to be vulnerable and ask for help. That wasn't always my strong suit, hey, love?' He squeezed Natalie's hand as best he could. 'Imagining dying is probably much scarier than actually dying. Does that make any sense?' he asked.

'It does to me. When we anticipate dying from the view of being in control, the thought of losing control gives rise to fear,' I replied. 'Our imagination instantly fills what precious time we have left with all sorts of scenarios, most of which will never happen. What *will* happen need not be feared. When we have little choice, and no control, conditioning takes over. But at a deeper level, our heart knows and understands what is happening and what to do. We just need a little reminding.'

'Yeah, it feels like some part of me knows how to do this,' John smiled.

Late one April afternoon I received a voicemail from Natalie.

'Will you come? John looks like he won't make it through the night.'

I let myself in the front door, slipped off my shoes and tiptoed through the kitchen to the den. A hospital bed had been set up there two weeks before, when John was finally too weak to climb the stairs. He wanted to be in the hub of the household, to be included in the family's activities – the mealtimes, the homework, the favourite TV shows.

Votive candles glowed along the windowsills and a wood fire burned low in the grate. Natalie was tucked into an armchair by the bed and the bedrail was lowered so she could hold John's hand.

'The kids just went to bed. I told them to. They

were tired.' She pointed to a chair by the fire. 'Pull it in close. Thanks for coming.'

The hollows under her eyes had deepened since my last visit. Neighbours and friends fetched groceries and cooked meals. Natalie told me she hadn't left the house for three days. Their daughter Mary had come home from university in the midst of her semester, and the other two hadn't wanted to go to school that week.

I leaned over to whisper in John's ear.

'Hi, John. I'll just sit here with Natalie to keep you both company for a bit. Hope that's okay.' I touched his forehead lightly and pushed a couple of stray hairs back into place along his hairline. I sat down beside Natalie and settled into the quiet of the vigil. We knew each other too well for small talk. We sat together for half an hour or so, listening to the oxygen flow into John's slowly failing lungs until Natalie tilted her head towards mine, keeping her eyes on John.

'It's almost over, isn't it? I think he's ready to go,' she murmured.

John's face was soft and relaxed, with no signs of pain or distress. His mouth was open and his breath was shallow and effortless. A light flow of oxygen entered his lungs through a tiny nasal cannula.

'You are helping him so much by creating such a

safe and loving atmosphere. He can rest in you and trust the process. It *is* almost over,' I replied.

'It feels like we've said everything there is to say. He knows how much I love him, and he knows that I'm not looking to replace him yet, right, honey?' She winked in John's direction. The absence of any flicker of response told me John was unconscious. He would likely die within hours.

'Don't be afraid to crawl in beside him. The bed's a bit narrow, but you'd fit,' I said.

Natalie nodded. 'I've wanted to do that, but have been scared it might hurt him.'

We dropped again into the quiet where time has no edges. I was there a good hour and everything felt settled. Rising from the chair, I leaned in closer to John.

'I'm heading home now. I'll keep a close eye on Natalie and the kids. They'll find a way through this together.' I kissed him lightly on the top of his head.

Reaching out my right hand to touch Natalie's arm, the cashmere was soft against the palm of my hand, and I could feel the warmth of life in her forearm beneath. She reached for a hug.

'Are you okay here by yourself tonight?' I asked.

'I think so. The kids told me that they don't want to be in the room at the end. That's okay, isn't it?' She looked at me.

'I trust kids to know what they need. If he does die tonight, you could wait until morning and then ask if they want to see him. Many kids want that, but it's best for them to decide. There's no need to rush after he dies. You will likely want time with him before he leaves the house.'

Natalie took my arm and walked me to the front hallway.

'How will I know when he's very close?' she asked.

'Do you notice how every few minutes there's a space of several seconds when John isn't breathing? Any time now, that pause will last longer. Eventually there will be one last breath,' I said.

Natalie nodded. 'Is that what's called apnoea, when there are spaces between the breaths?'

'It is,' I said. 'I often wonder what it's like to dwell in that place of no breath, before returning to breathing again. I imagine it as a different plane of consciousness not understood by our minds. Perhaps it's like travelling to a new country a few times before you decide to make it your home.'

'I like the thought that it might be okay to die, that there is an energy that carries on after the body dies,' Natalie said. 'John never believed anything like that, but I like to think that his spirit will dissolve into a vast space of love.'

'I like to think of it that way too,' I said.

At times, it seems to me as if the spirit reveals its presence as death approaches. If we focus only on the weakening body as it changes colour and temperature, as it emits a sour or sweet odour that comes from shallow, slow or rapid breathing, or produces sounds of grunting or moaning or incomprehensible words, we might miss an almost imperceptible energy that radiates from soft eyes, or through translucent skin. We may fail to notice that the room itself compels a reverence.

However, sometimes the grief is too vast to put our attention on anything other than who and what we are losing, what we will miss, how we will cope. Sometimes we can only hope that if there is a spirit, it will know what to do when we are too bereft to notice.

I did sense an energy that evening in the room with John and Natalie, that was unaffected by the dying of his physical body, a presence that calmed me and helped me to trust the dying process implicitly. My heartbreak that night was for Natalie and the three children sleeping, or trying to sleep, upstairs.

Natalie and I hugged for what we both knew would be the last time while John was alive. I let myself out of the front door and breathed in the sharp cold of the deep indigo night.

John died between two and two-thirty that morning. Natalie called me at eight to tell me she had fallen asleep in the bed with her arm across his chest. He took his last breath while she slept. The only sound she heard when she awoke was the gentle hiss of the oxygen.

5

DAN: Dying on His
Own Terms

Tina handed me a red playing card on which was
a small black-and-white headshot of a man in a
fedora and sunglasses. The words *the DANNY card* were
printed across it. I turned the card over and read:

Abilities: 1. Never stop asking yourself, 'Who
                 am I?'
              2. Be honest with yourself and others.
              3. Passionately pursue things you
                 care about.
              4. Value community, friends and
                 family.

Methods   1. *The Danny*: Play in support
of Play: of another player.
              2. *The Self-Danny*: Play to support
                 yourself.

Dylan had designed the cards for his brother Dan's Celebration of Life, which was held three days before the day Dan had chosen to die. Medical Assistance in Dying (MAID) had become legal in Canada a year before.

'All eighty of us were given a card to take home,' Tina said, as she and I sat together in my office two months later. She'd come from work at the end of her day and told me that going back to work had been a helpful distraction from her grief, even though the nights were hard. 'Without Dan at our backs now, with his unshakeable faith in us making the world a better place, Dylan thought we needed this card as a reminder,' she said.

You might pull the card out of your pocket and *Danny* your spouse if he or she is grumpy or out-of-sorts, or if you need a kick in the pants you can *Danny* yourself into action. Dan, affectionately known as Guru Dan, had spent much of his thirty-six years of life inspiring family and friends to do their personal growth work, like he had, to become forces for good in the world. The *Danny* card was intended to be a talisman for the continued presence of Guru Dan in their lives.

Born in 1981, Dan had sixteen healthy years before being diagnosed with FAP (familial adenomatous polyposis), an inherited disease of the colon causing severe abdominal pain and bowel obstructions. Dan spent the next fifteen years improving his health through diet, exercise and personal growth courses, but eventually, in December 2010, when he was twenty-nine years old, Dan opted for the extensive surgery known as the Whipple procedure to remove his duodenum, gallbladder and the head of his pancreas, with the intention of removing a multitude of polyps which had a 99 per cent chance of becoming cancerous.

Around 10–20 per cent of people with FAP also go on to develop desmoid tumours, which although benign cause serious and life-threatening problems. Dan developed these tumours one year after the Whipple surgery, requiring him to have another operation to remove his entire colon. In the autumn of 2015, Dan almost died from a haemorrhage and spent most of the next two months in and out of intensive care. After recovering enough to go home, he suffered a series of life-threatening infections that forced him back to hospital many times over the next seven months, and by the time we met, Dan had undergone nine surgeries and survived only because of perpetual courses of antibiotics and intravenous feeding (Total Parenteral Nutrition: TPN). In his last meeting with the surgeon a month before we met, Dan was told there were no more surgical options. Soon after, he began conversations with his wife, family and GP about MAID.

* * *

Dan called our office in early February 2017 and asked to talk to a counsellor about 'dying with dignity'. For Dan, dying with dignity meant activating his legal right to choose to die with the assistance of a physician. He came to the first counselling session with his wife Tina and his brother Dylan.

Once comfortable on the couch with several pillows propped at his back, I asked Dan to tell me his story. His weary gaze conveyed a man tired of telling the details of his difficult life to yet another healthcare professional who may or may not be able to help. Dan took a deep breath and began, pausing here and there for a breath, or for Tina or Dylan to fill in details so he could rest for a few moments. He told me he was in constant pain, suffered debilitating fatigue and continued to lose weight despite being on TPN. He took me through a litany of traumatic encounters. Each one had required him to surrender his ailing body to a healthcare system that would inevitably fall short of solutions.

Dan's fatigue infused the sound of every word, flattening out its tone, like when the overplayed strings of a guitar lose their pitch. He was thorough in his storytelling, wanting me to understand that he had reached the end of the road and that life could no longer serve his dreams and passions. He explained that if there had been any more options he'd have kept fighting, but there weren't and so he would learn to accept his dying, and help his family and friends to accept it too.

Tina and Dylan listened to Dan speak attentively, their capacity to lift him back up into life long past. Dylan described the elaborate spreadsheet of questions and concerns that Dan presented at each doctor's appointment.

'The physician often deferred to Dan, saying that he knew more than the doctors did,' Dylan said. 'Dan always asked, "Have you seen this before?" or "Is this normal?". Once an engineer, always an engineer. We are excellent problem-solvers.'

Dan spoke of his determination not to die in a hospital, a place where he had spent too many days and weeks already. 'I'm basically tired of being a medical experiment,' he said. 'I want control over the end, not to die attached to tubes and machines in a hospital. Thank God MAID is available or I don't know what I'd do.' He looked up at me with a questioning look, as though gauging where I stood on the issue.

'You are taking charge of the end of your life with the same kind of tenacity with which you have tackled your life. No one really understands how much you are suffering except for you, and perhaps Tina, who is with you most moments of your days and nights.

Trust yourself to do what's right.' Dan glanced at Tina, whose face crumpled at the memories of nights changing sweat-soaked bed linens, and her hopes for pain relief that evaporated with each renewed spasm. Watching the one you love the most suffer, and not be able to help, is a torture all of its own.

Dan continued to empty out the stories of his life, as if he had been waiting for a long time to speak them collectively as one story. Tina nodded and encouraged him to go on when he faltered, an occasional tear quickly wiped away from her cheek. After about forty minutes, Dan had caught up with the present and I then directed my attention to a time before many of the traumatic stories happened. I wanted to know who Dan was before his illness took charge.

'What do you miss most about yourself?' I asked.

'I miss the adventures, the travelling, just doing stuff with friends,' Dan said. 'We lived and worked in Thailand for two years. It was amazing.' Dan grabbed Tina's hand and glanced at her, nostalgia rimming his eyes, then quickly turned away before the emotion could take full hold. 'And I miss the garden. Do you know the Green Guys on The Drive?' he asked. I shook my head, no.

'After I decided I didn't want to be an engineer any more, I started a business with my best friend. We wanted to show people how to grow their own veggies locally even from a downtown apartment.' Dan smiled with pride. 'We started the first community-supported vertical hydroponic urban vegetable farm,' he said, with a small burst of energy brightening his eyes. 'We wanted to create a community for ourselves. It was really, really important to us and it worked.'

Dan dropped his head towards his lap and paused. I could feel the ending that was upon him; the end of a life of purpose and vision, a life with no more options, and a life that required energy he no longer had.

'I can't do it any more,' Dan whispered, looking up at Tina.

'I know,' she said. 'I don't need you to have to.'

A couple of weeks later, Dan and Tina met with two separate MAID assessors, who ascertained whether Dan fit the criteria for MAID: 1. Being at least eighteen years old and capable of making his own healthcare decisions; 2. Having a serious and incurable illness in an advanced state of irreversible decline; 3. Having enduring and intolerable suffering that cannot be relieved by any means acceptable to the patient; 4. Death has become reasonably foreseeable; 5. Making a voluntary request for MAID that is not the result of outside pressure or influence; 6. Giving consent to receive MAID after being provided with all the information necessary to make the decision; 7. Being eligible for publicly funded health services in Canada. Dan satisfied the criteria and the paperwork was completed. He decided that MAID would happen sometime in April. He was still to pick a date.

I was away for a couple of weeks, during which time Dan called and asked if he and his father could come for counselling. He had several topics he wanted to talk with his dad about and thought it would be helpful to have a third person present for the conversation. One of my counselling colleagues was able to see them and Dan told me that the session had helped him to be honest with his father. 'I am at peace now with the past, with everything,' he said.

'How is he with your MAID decision?' I asked.

'He struggled at first with it. Who wouldn't try to stop your son from dying? But now he accepts my decision and will be there for me when the time comes.'

'What about your mother?' I asked, as he hadn't mentioned his mom.

'Sadly, she has dementia, and I can't tell her my plans until closer to the time as it will be hard for her to understand and it will totally upset her.'

Dan told me he planned to meet with his mother

a week or so before the date he chose for MAID and try to explain his decision to her.

The next time I saw Dan was a month after our first session. He came with his brother Dylan and they talked for two hours about their complex and intimate life as brothers. They reviewed their life together, their ups and downs, and I could feel the form and shape of their memories holding them together. I sensed that for Dylan this conversation would be a balm for his grief later, when their brotherly relationship would get redefined in Dan's absence. The love continues after someone we love dies, especially when we are unencumbered with wishes for conversations that never happened.

I remember pausing to watch the brothers leave the building that day, their continuing discussion floating in through the open window as they went down the outside stairs. As they crossed the street, Dylan slung his arm over Dan's bony frame and pulled him into his chest. They had started the process of saying goodbye.

I felt such gratitude for the courage these two brothers had for this conversation, one that many families choose not to have because it requires a willingness to be vulnerable. Family members often worry that engaging in talk about dying with their loved ones might be perceived as them giving up hope. This fear often becomes regret for the family members later. Dying people often want to protect their loved ones from the hurt of separation and choose to avoid talking about it. Both Dan and Dylan were up for having the hardest conversations.

Dan was diligent in tending to his family and friends, and it took every ounce of the little energy he had left. He was specifically building and maintaining community around him, not just to support him in his own last weeks or months, but to set the practices in place for the people he would leave behind, showing them how to be vulnerable and talk to one another, paving the way for healthy grieving. Many dying people become isolated from their community at the end of life because they don't know how to stay connected. They don't know how to ask for help. Dan was a master at both.

The last time I saw Dan was when he came to see me with Tina to talk about moving forward with a date for MAID, and to go over their final preparations. It had been a month since I had last seen him, and though physically weaker, he had the clarity of a man who had done his work. He came in with an agenda.

'I want a going-away party while I'm still alive, not a funeral afterwards,' he said. 'Probably eighty or so people. Family and friends. My dad will speak, and Dylan, and I hope I can say a few words too. I can't last much longer.'

Dan set the date for the party, three days before he would die, and ten days from our last meeting. He arranged with a friend to use her apartment, as Tina did not want the memory of his death to be imprinted in their bed and their home. He invited more than twenty people to be present with him at his death.

'What do you think happens after death?' Dan asked me out of the blue that day. 'I'm asking everyone what they think because I don't know what I believe.'

'I don't know either,' I said, 'but my work, with dying children especially, helps me to believe that there is an energy that continues on after our bodies die.' I told Dan stories of children who talked to me about the places they were going in such exquisite detail and with such enthusiasm that it was difficult to refute that there is a spirit, an individual energy that merges with consciousness after we take our last breath. Their faith was compelling.

'Say more,' Dan said.

'I've also had several experiences in meditation over the years, especially on longer retreats, of an awareness that the body seems to have no edges, and that form itself is an illusion. I find these states interesting, but at the end of the day I'm living, not dying, and death is really still a mystery, isn't it?' I asked.

Dan nodded. 'I don't have much faith in an after-life, though I wish I did.'

I was aware that the date Dan had alluded to in our last visit was looming but I hadn't heard that it had been confirmed. I lit a candle beside my desk that day and thought of Dan, and Tina and Dylan and the community around them, and I hoped that his death was just as he had envisioned. A few days passed and I hadn't heard any news so I decided to contact Tina. I only had Dan's cellphone number, so I dialled, thinking there would be no answer, or that Tina might pick up. To my surprise I heard Dan's voice at the end of the phone. 'Hey,' he said.

'It's Janie here. I wasn't expecting you to pick up.'

'Why not?'

'I thought you might already be gone,' I said awkwardly, not knowing if he had perhaps changed his mind, or something else had happened and he had ended up in hospital.

'It's on Saturday,' he said.

'Oh . . . right. How are you feeling about every-thing?' I asked.

'I feel settled,' Dan said. 'I know this is the right thing, and thanks by the way for all your help.'

'You did the work, Dan. I've learned a lot from you, and I respect you and your family so much for being so conscious and loving throughout this whole process. I will be surrounding you from a distance on Saturday with my love.'

'Bye,' he said simply, and hung up the phone.

I had never had a conversation like this before with a dying person. There had never been a 'known' time that death would for sure occur. There is always a mystery that the uncertainty of the time of death brings, and a period of vigil where I go through my days in a kind of sacred holding, until the news is shared that the person has died. I like to think of the holding as a kind of prayer for ease and peace in those last moments of life.

I was very touched when Tina said she thought Dan would like to have his story written in this book. 'He always was such a public guy, and his choice in dying was no exception. He told anyone who would listen that this was what he was going to do. It's all about community with Dan,' she said.

When she arrived at my office just a few weeks after his death, she looked more rested than when I had seen her before. In the first month or two of bereavement the psyche is protective, helping to keep some of the more intense emotions below the surface, until later. This mechanism helps people to function in their activities of daily living, which helps to assuage the loneliness and sadness that inevitably permeates in due course.

I asked Tina if she could tell me about the last days of Dan's life. She described the party for eighty people and said she would bring me a video, if I was interested. I said, 'Of course.'

On the day of Dan's death, the group of about twenty-five people took a slow walk to a nearby beach where three friends played guitars and they sang old favourites. After half an hour or so, they strolled back to the apartment where everyone then sat in a circle in the living room, and each person had a chance to speak to Dan. 'There was not a dry eye in the house,' Tina said. A ceremony was then performed with Dan and Tina lying on a blanket and the group lifted and rocked them while the song 'I Want To Live' played in the background. It was a ceremony that Dan had learned about in one of the personal growth courses he had attended a few years before. Tina described how peaceful Dan felt throughout the ceremony.

In the bedroom, Tina was aware that the team of two doctors (one MAID provider and one in training) and one nurse were quietly setting up for the procedure. When Dan was ready he lay down on the bed while Tina and Dylan sat on the bed beside him.

The doctor described to Dan what medications he would receive, first a drug to relax and sedate him, second an anaesthesia drug to induce coma, and third a neuromuscular blocker. She then asked Dan if he wished to go ahead, obtaining final consent for the procedure. Before he told them to begin, Dan described the procedure in depth to the group standing in a circle around his bed. He wished for them all to be at peace with his choice even if it wasn't their preference. He then chose to have a final moment outside on the balcony in the fresh air with Tina, Dylan and his father before proceeding. When Dan lay back down on the bed the physician infused the three different medications into Dan's IV. Within a few moments Dan went into a deep sleep, and at the end of the final drug infusion the doctor said, 'His heart has stopped. It is completed.'

Tina described how everyone hugged and cried after it was over, and within ten minutes or so they left the apartment to have dinner together in a nearby restaurant. Dylan and a friend stayed with Dan for around two hours until the funeral home arrived to transport Dan's body. They then joined the group at the restaurant.

Tina told me she felt such comfort knowing that the group had gone through Dan's death together, as a community, just as Dan had wanted.

In the year following Dan's death, the community gathered several times and no one expressed regret or concern around Dan's choice. They felt only honour at being included in such a peaceful and dignified death, and glad that Dan had died on his own terms.

II.

ACCEPTING THE
UNRESOLVED HEART

*'Have patience with everything
unresolved in your heart'*
—RAINER MARIA RILKE

Like the birth process, dying does not always unfold in the way we hope or plan for. Even with forethought and preparation, dying is rarely predictable. Pain can be hard to manage, unforeseen family dynamics arise, personalities become unrecognisable, unrealistic hopes surface, expectations shatter and unresolved feelings can lodge for a lifetime.

In death, family relationships can be as complicated as in life, and discord at the end of life has little chance of being resolved because the opportunity for further conversation has passed. How do we deal with our guilt and regret after a loved one dies, or hold questions that we know can never be answered? Often the most we can hope for is that, over months or years, with patience, we can come to accept what is unresolved in our hearts and make peace with the experience, however difficult and life-altering it was.

Most families hold complex and difficult stories about death which inform and shape their feelings, attitudes, beliefs and choices about mortality. Our stories and experiences directly affect our personal choices in living and dying, which in turn deeply affect the people we love. The four stories in *Accepting the Unresolved Heart* describe people grappling with the complexity of relationships, decisions and choices, exploring the ethics and moral distress in relation to their own death, or the dying of another person.

6

BRIGID: Best Laid Plans

'He'd cryopreserve me if he could,' Brigid said with a nervous chuckle. She had asked to talk privately with me about some 'family matters' one afternoon during a weeklong retreat for alumni. I met Brigid when she had attended a retreat two years earlier, and since that time she was a regular member in the support groups at our centre.

Brigid's reddish-blonde wig was made from real hair, styled into a bob with a fringe. She said she paid a fortune for it, and it was scratchy as hell, but her husband Colin preferred her to wear the wig when they went out in public. She'd go out bald if it wasn't for him, a badge of honour, she said, for all the chemotherapy she had tolerated. This was a second marriage for them both and they had hoped for a lot more years together. Colin had just retired and they had made plans to travel when Brigid finished up work in two years, with a full pension from the School Board. The Galapagos had been the first destination on their bucket list.

'He said he couldn't live with his loneliness if I died.' Brigid took a deep breath. 'I said to him, "Honey, it's not if, but when."'

I nodded. 'The people who love us want to believe we'll live for ever.' I felt Brigid's pragmatism bump up against Colin's need to deny the reality of losing her, at least for a while. She would need to be patient, and I sensed that patience might not be one of her virtues.

Brigid's liver housed her third recurrence of cancer and she was determined to be at peace at the end of her life. There's often hope for a cure when breast cancer is first diagnosed, but if it recurs, a different kind of reality settles in: the cancer shifts from being curable to incurable. The first time Brigid was diagnosed with breast cancer five years before her first retreat, she thought she would just have to endure the surgery, radiation and chemotherapy, and then she would be cured. She assumed that her one brush with cancer would be her last. When she learned that the cancer had spread to her bones, three years after the initial cancer, she was shocked. Her oncologist told her that even with chemotherapy, the cancer would keep coming back. She might get some months, even a year or two between bouts, but she wouldn't ever be cured. She got twenty months between the second and third recurrences. Brigid hoped her acceptance of death would eventually rub off on Colin because she knew that she would likely not get a third remission or a fourth recurrence.

'My parents both died of old age in their nineties, in their own bed, my father seven years before my mother. They were farmers and understood the cycle of life and death. They weren't afraid of death,' she said.

Her Irish lineage imbued Brigid with fortitude, built on generations of men and women who cared for dying loved ones at home, strength she hoped to draw upon when her time came.

'My sisters and brothers nursed Mummy and Dad, and I went home for a few weeks. No muss or fuss, just a gentle fading away. That's how I want it to be for me, if possible. No keeping me alive when it's clear I'm done.'

Brigid's pale green eyes drifted off into the distance for a moment, before she spoke again.

'Now I have to convince Colin I could die at home,' she said. 'I have a big task ahead of me.'

Both Colin's parents had died in hospital. His father had a heart attack on the golf course at fifty-eight and was rushed to hospital, where he died a week later in the coronary care unit. His mother was in her mid-seventies when she fell at home and died in Emergency. Brigid told me Colin thought he should have done more to prevent his parents from dying, such as insist his father have a cardiac check-up even though he had no history of angina, or set up more help for his mum at home. He hadn't accepted that he had little control over their deaths.

'Colin can't stand hearing the word *palliative* when my doctor or nurse refers to me that way,' Brigid said.

'Most people get scared when they hear the word *palliative*, because they assume it means death is imminent,' I said. Brigid knew that becoming palliative meant that the focus of medical care had changed from curing her cancer to treating the symptoms of her disease to maximise her quality of life. Studies have shown that early referral to palliative care not only helps people to live better, it can also lead to living longer. Researchers have surmised that better symptom management creates a short-term stability in the patient's medical condition, and hence fewer acute life-threatening occurrences. Colin either thought the term 'palliative' meant Brigid's death was imminent, or, more likely, any word that pointed to her certain death terrified him.

'I think my quality of life is pretty good, except I tire easily. I can't do as much as I used to and my garden has certainly suffered without me. Will I get more and more tired as I get closer?' Brigid asked.

'You'll have diminishing energy as time goes on, and you'll want to rest more. When your liver isn't working, toxins build up in your system and cause fatigue. Not easy for someone like you, I imagine?' I said.

'I've never been good at doing nothing. Colin is always after me to come in from the garden, but it helps me to know that the bulbs I planted will be there for him in the spring, even if I'm not.' She looked down at her rugged gardener's hands. 'He hates it when I talk like this,' she said. Irritation nipped at the edges of her words.

She was afraid to tell her husband she wanted her ashes scattered in the garden, like good mulch, and that she wanted a 'proper' funeral, not a celebration of life where no one is allowed to cry. She told me that the Irish believe in mourning properly, with the help of a few whiskies, and that after the service the bereaved should get on with life, make the best of it. Her voice carried the melancholy of belonging to two countries within one life.

'I've tried to talk about it,' she said. 'But he just tells me it's not going to happen.' Brigid looked off into the distance. Colin's resistance had wedged a cold stone of loneliness into her heart.

In the silence that followed, we both waited for the other to speak first. Finally, Brigid turned her head to face me. 'Can you tell me what it's going to be like at the end, how I'll die?'

'Most likely the cancer in your liver will be the main problem. When the liver fails, dying is usually a gentle process over a few days, or up to two or three weeks.' Brigid's gaze was unflinching as I explained how she would become more and more sleepy, and near the very end she would sleep most of the day, as well as the night. The last days would be comfortable as long as she had the medications she needed for symptoms such as pain or nausea.

'There is often more peace in the room if family and friends accept you're dying,' I said.

'Colin can't accept it.' Brigid clenched her bony hands together. 'I don't know what to do.'

'Have you been able to talk to him about a DNAR?' I asked, referring to the Do Not Attempt Resuscitation document that informs a person's healthcare team about their wishes. 'Most of us don't wish for heroic measures then.'

'I've got the form in my purse, signed, but I've been too scared to tell Colin,' she said.

The home care nurse had told Brigid to tape the

paperwork to the fridge in the kitchen, so that if Colin got frightened and called an ambulance the paramedics would see the form and know not to resuscitate Brigid and put her on life support. Without a signed form, they would be required by law to resuscitate her.

The wind rattled against the large-paned windows of the group room. It was late October, and the snow would be on its way soon. There were just a few leaves clinging to bare branches, waiting for the next gust of wind to take them. The earth doesn't have to prepare for the changing seasons like people do.

'That brings me to the subject of your Advanced Directive. If you become unable to make medical decisions, you can legally designate someone else to make those decisions for you,' I said.

Brigid leaned forward onto the edge of her seat. 'Colin is not the right person to be my medical representative. Even though I've told him my wishes, I don't think he could follow them. He wants me here at any cost.' She fidgeted as she spoke and her head bobbed anxiously from side to side.

'Choosing someone else to make those decisions for you might relieve Colin of a responsibility that is too hard for him,' I said. Brigid's facial muscles softened on Colin's behalf.

'My best friend would be a better choice. She wouldn't be afraid to pull the plug,' Brigid said.

'I wonder if Colin would be open to meeting with Daphne, our retreat physician? You will have a medical session with her tomorrow?' I said, thinking that Daphne, with twenty-five years of palliative care experience talking with family members, might be able to ease Colin's fears and help him to come to terms with the situation.

'I could ask him,' she said. 'If anyone could get through to him, it might be someone like Daphne.'

A couple of months later, Brigid called me from the hospital. She told me she had a high fever and was having trouble breathing. Colin had wanted to take her to Emergency in the middle of the night, but she refused to go until the morning. Her oncologist was away on vacation, so she had seen an internist who told her she had pneumonia.

'My breathing is much worse since being admitted yesterday,' she whispered, between pauses for air. 'Do you think this might be it, Janie?'

'It might be, but there is a chance that the antibiotics will work. Do you want me to ask if you could be admitted to the palliative care unit?' I asked.

'Yes, but Colin refuses to have me go there. The doctor says that if my breathing gets any worse today, they could admit me to intensive care to be ventilated on a machine. They think if I have a few days in there, with the machine breathing for me and antibiotics, then maybe I'll be okay.' Her voice shook.

'You can receive IV antibiotics on the palliative care unit without having to be intubated with a ventilator breathing for you,' I said. 'The antibiotics will either work or they won't, and the two environments couldn't be more different: being ventilated in the ICU means you'd be sedated and wouldn't be able to talk to Colin, who would be one of the few visitors allowed; in the PCU you wouldn't be attached to machines, nor sedated, and you could have as many visitors as you like. Do you know what you want to do, Brigid?' I asked softly.

'No, not really,' she said.

As long as Brigid was conscious, she would be in charge of her healthcare decisions, but as soon as she lost consciousness Colin would make decisions for her, as her next-of-kin, unless she had designated her best friend to be her medical representative.

'Did you and Colin ever complete the paperwork for your Advanced Directive?' I asked, already suspecting what her answer would be.

'I asked him this past weekend but he was adamant about not meeting a palliative care doctor yet. He kept saying he'd never give up on me. And Janie, I hate to admit it, but I was too scared to tell him that

I trust my friend more than him to make decisions on my behalf.' Brigid's voice was resigned.

'Would you be able to talk to Colin and the doctor now to explain your wishes?' I heard the urgency in my own voice. Brigid only had a small window of time before decisions would be out of her hands.

'Can I call you later?' she said.

'Of course, and I can come and help with the conversation, if you want me to,' I said.

'Thanks, Janie. I'll keep you posted.'

The call from Brigid never came. The following morning, I phoned the hospital to see if I could locate her. I was told she was in intensive care and no visitors were allowed, except close family.

I left a voicemail for Colin at home, the only phone number I had for him.

'Colin, I heard Brigid is in intensive care. I am so sorry. Would you call me back?' I left my cellphone number.

He didn't call.

Brigid died two weeks later. I read her obituary in our local newspaper:

After a valiant battle with cancer, Brigid O'Sullivan died in the intensive care unit at Vancouver General Hospital . . . her beloved husband Colin was at her side.

7

JIM: No Talk of Dying

Shona MacKenzie left me a voicemail in a Scottish brogue almost too thick to understand, although hearing a Glaswegian speak always lifts my spirits.

When I returned Shona's call, she told me she'd been given my name by her husband's home care nurse.

'The nurse thought you might be able to knock some sense into my husband's head,' she said.

'What's happening?' I asked.

'He thinks he's getting out on the golf course again, but he's kidding himself! He's far too sick now for golf,' Shona said. 'We've a lot to sort out but he won't talk.'

'Does Jim know you've called me?'

'I've not told him yet. He's not one for counselling.'

'Is anyone in Scotland into counselling?' I laughed.

'You're right, lass. A pint of beer is a better solution to emotional problems,' Shona said.

'Tell Jim you've invited me for tea, and that I'm from the old country,' I said. 'He might let me in the door then.'

Whenever I drive to North Vancouver, I turn right just before the causeway to the Lions Gate Bridge so I can go the long way around, through Stanley Park. The giant Douglas firs and Western red cedars lining the edge of the road that loops through the park steady me somehow. I once asked an Indigenous friend about the big trees, how they must have so much energy, or life force, to be able to withstand gales and snowstorms, given that their root system is relatively shallow.

'Pity we can't harness the energy of the great trees for ourselves, or for people who need strength,' I had said to my friend Bev.

'Of course you can,' she replied briskly.

'How?' I asked.

'Just ask them for some energy, and then thank them. They never say no.' She laughed.

As I drove around the park with the trees on my left that day, the spring sunshine illuminated the white sails of the Pan Pacific Hotel and bounced off the high-rises that delineate the cityscape. I could see the mounds of bright yellow sulphur on the far shore of Burrard Inlet and the last small patches of snow on the North Shore Mountains.

I pulled up outside a white-sided bungalow tucked in under the mountain. Firs and cedars were there too, at the back of the property, and being a few minutes early I sat in the car, closed my eyes and asked for strength from them, making sure I said aloud, 'Thank you.'

I walked down the path to the house and knocked on the weathered front door. Shona was just as I had imagined her to be from her voice on the phone: in her early seventies, with permed sandy-grey hair cut to just above the collar of her blue cotton blouse. She wore a small gold cross on a chain around her neck, tucked inside her top. Her wide-legged polyester trousers were cinched in at the waist with a navy belt and her flat open-toed sandals were worn with socks.

'Thanks for coming.' I held out my hand to shake her cool and slightly clammy hand, and I thought maybe she was nervous too. Meeting a family for the first time often causes me anxiety, as establishing rapport quickly is essential in order to be useful. Entering a family's home at such a sensitive time feels like a privilege, one you are frequently not sure you have earned.

'I will take you right in to see Jim, but he's not feeling so good today,' Shona whispered. 'He was awake most of the night in a sweat and he's not eaten much in the last few days. The doctor is coming later to check on him.'

Shona went ahead of me into the small bedroom, with its hospital bed pushed up against a double bed. Every surface was covered with trinkets: miniature china dogs and plastic ballerinas, wind-up music boxes and dusty wooden nativity scenes. Framed black-and-white photographs of historic sites of Scotland dotted the walls and the curtains were closed against the sun trying to shine through the crack between. Jim was propped up with several pillows and he wore a pair of blue-striped pyjamas, buttoned up to the collar. His damp hair was combed neatly over to one side. Shona would likely have freshened him up after his rough night to receive a visitor.

'Jim, this is Janie, the nurse I told you was coming for tea,' she said.

I held out my hand and felt a good strong hand-shake returned.

'Good afternoon,' Jim said. 'Sorry to be meeting in here, but I had a bad night. I'll be up and about later.' Shona stole a glance at me and raised her eyebrows.

'Good to meet you,' I said. 'I'll stay for as long as you're up for it.'

'Up for what?' he asked, his dark shaggy eyebrows rising with the question.

'Shona phoned me to see if I could come and meet you, to see if I could help,' I said.

'Help with what? I don't need a shrink, if that's what you are. I just need to get out on the course and hit a few balls.'

I sat down on the chair Shona must have placed at the side of the bed for me. She was perched on a stool at the foot, her legs crossed at the knee, and one sandal wagged up and down in an agitated way. Shona had an agenda.

'Jim, darlin', be nice! Janie is a nurse, and she's from Glasgow,' Shona said, patting his foot under the quilt.

'I won't hold that against you,' Jim said. 'Not your fault.' He winked.

'My dad was born and raised in Ayr, though. Does that help?' I asked.

'That's near Largs, where we're both from. Is your dad a golfer?'

I knew I'd score some points on the golf. 'He was a golfer, got his handicap down to nine in his best years, and my mum, she lives in Glasgow and still golfs at eighty-six. Dad died almost twenty years ago.'

'What did he die of, if you don't mind me asking?' Jim said.

'A brain tumour. Stage IV when he was diagnosed, out of the blue.'

'My lung cancer's Stage IV too, and I hear there's no Stage V.' He looked at me while boxing the air with both fists. 'I'm a fighter, though, so it's not going to take me out for a good long while.'

I noticed Jim's pale blue nails and how his chest moved with effort for every breath. I wondered how long it would be until he needed an oxygen tank.

Shona slid her agenda into the conversation.

'Jimmy, that's not what the doctor said last week. She said she couldn't give you any more chemo, and she was sorry.'

'Get Janie some tea, darlin'. She doesn't want to hear you being so negative.' Jim shooed her away with a flick of his bony wrist.

He started speaking as soon as Shona slipped into the kitchen.

'I'm worried about her. What's she going to do when I'm dead? She's not well herself, and the kids are too busy to look in on her. I've taken care of the money side of things, so that's good,' Jim said.

I took the opportunity while I could. 'It'll be hard on her, no question. You can't protect her from her sadness, though, and she's probably stronger than you think.'

'She thinks I don't understand how sick I am, but I do. I just think it's better not to talk about it. Gets her all upset.' He dragged his hand through his hair and held on to the back of his neck. 'When she gets upset, then I cannae hold it together.'

'It might help her if you could talk about it,' I said.

'I don't know what to say,' he said. He seemed like a man who had relied on his physical and mental strength, but with his diminishing stamina and lowered ability to provide for and protect his wife, he wasn't sure how to adjust to his increasing dependency and the accompanying feelings that were just below the surface.

'Here we go!' Shona announced, carrying a tray of teacups and saucers, a sugar bowl and milk jug, a classic Brown Betty teapot swathed in a knitted tea-cosy, and a plate of chocolate digestive biscuits. She set the tray down on the bed, the only clear surface in the room.

'What do you take in your tea, Janie?'

'Just milk, thanks.'

She poured the milk in first and then tipped steaming tea into the cup, to the brim.

'Do you want some tea, Jim?' she asked.

'No thanks, darlin'. I'm already burning up.'

'What did you two get to talking about in my absence?' Shona asked. Jim looked at me and raised his eyebrows.

'We talked about the weather. How mild it is for spring,' he said.

I sipped my tea. 'Is there anything either of you want to talk about, or ask me, while I'm here?'

They looked at each other, waiting to see if the other would respond.

Shona tried again. 'Jim, I want to talk to Janie about what's going to happen when you get sicker.'

'What about it?' he asked, his protective armour moving into place.

'Are you going to want to be at the hospice, or stay here?' she asked.

'How many times do I have to tell you, I'm still planning to play another round of golf or two before I kick the bucket. Let's talk about this another time,' Jim said, the frown line between his brows deepening. 'Whereabouts in Glasgow are you from, Janie?'

I visited Jim and Shona three weeks later in Lions Gate Hospital. She had phoned and asked me to come. Jim's fever hadn't responded to antibiotics, and he was confused. His lungs were congested and he required high-flow oxygen. When Shona suggested he go into the hospice, he said no, but he did let her take him to Emergency. He still talked about getting out for nine holes, in the few lucid moments he had. Shona told me on the phone that Jim still refused to talk about dying, or have his will drawn up. He wouldn't sign the Do Not Attempt Resuscitation paperwork, which meant he couldn't be considered for the hospice. She had finally given up trying to get him to open up. I could see the pain in her eyes of the surrender, of giving up the potential for a verbal goodbye.

I entered the four-bed room and saw that Jim was asleep in the bed by the window. Shona slouched in an armchair pulled up as close as possible to the bed.

'Sit over there, Janie.' Shona pointed to a chair on the other side of the bed. 'Jim, Janie's here, remember that lassie who came to see us at home?' she said loudly, leaning towards his left ear, but there was no sign that he had registered Shona's words, or my presence.

'It's been terrible. He's been frantic, and restless, shouting out. He scared the kids off yesterday with his ranting and I told them to go home for a rest,' she said. 'Finally, the nurse asked me about sedation, used to calm people who are suffering too much, and I said, "Yes, do it."' Jim continued to sleep as we talked.

'When oxygen levels fall very low, people often become confused, and being a Scot, I am not surprised his fighting instinct kicked in,' I said. I went on to explain that when survival is threatened, a person feels out of control and defaults to habitual ways of reacting: we fight, run away, freeze or surrender. The continuous sedation he received through the intravenous infusion helped Jim to surrender and, three days after my visit to the hospital, he died.

'I guess he couldn't accept he was dying,' Shona said, in a counselling session two weeks later. 'Is that what the "death and dying" books call denial?' she asked.

'To be honest, Shona, I don't believe there's such a thing as denial in dying,' I replied. 'I think Jim made a choice to keep his thoughts and feelings to himself, not out of malevolence, but out of care for you. He thought it would upset you too much.'

Shona reached for the little gold cross under her blouse and rubbed it between her forefinger and thumb.

'It felt like we were pretending when he talked about getting back to golf. I'm so mad at him for not being braver, and not talking to me about the fact he was dying.'

I nodded. 'Fear of feeling the sadness of saying goodbye was likely too much for him,' I said.

'Except after a few pints; then he's maudlin,' she said, and sighed. 'I'm mostly sad we didn't get to say goodbye,' she sniffed. 'I miss that stubborn old bugger. I really do.'

8

PAT: The Decision

'Everyone tells me to keep fighting, to never give up hope,' Pat said with a shrug of her emaciated shoulders. 'Is dying about giving up hope? Is it really a choice? I'm confused.'

We sat on the loveseat facing the small living-room window of her basement flat, our knees almost touching. The evergreen magnolia peeked over the sill with its shiny dark green leaves with brown undersides. Pat loved her garden. She'd owned a gardening business but by age forty-one, when she was first diagnosed with a rare cancer of the appendix, she was onto her fifth career, as a computer programmer for a funeral company.

'Healthy people can tell me to stay hopeful, but try living in this body. Nine years of cancer. I never expected to make it to fifty and now I'm fifty-one,'

Pat said. 'Has it been the fighting that has kept me here this long, or is it just the way the disease goes, fight or no fight? Everyone assumes that all I have to do is try harder and I'll live longer. I reckon I've just been very lucky, and now my time's running out.' Pat looked down, pondering her own enquiry. She lifted her head up and changed the subject. 'What have you been up to? Saving all the poor souls like me? You should get a life!' she laughed.

Earlier that day, Pat had called me. She had been second-guessing the decision to have surgery and wanted to talk it over. We had known each other for six years by then. After her first retreat, Pat became a volunteer at Callanish, helping in the office whenever she had the energy. We loved having her around, with her lightness of being and brilliant sense of humour. The cancer now pushed against her spinal column, causing excruciating pain and weakness in her legs. Walking had become difficult, and Pat relied on her home support worker for bathing, dressing, cooking and cleaning. Her independence was rapidly deteriorating.

'Do my friends and family think it will be my fault if I die? Maybe they don't want to accept that getting cancer is random, that it could happen to them too.'

Pat looked up at me and I nodded.

The surgeon had booked the surgery. He told her

he could operate to try to remove the tumour near her spine. Without surgery, there was a fifty-fifty chance that the growing cancer would destroy enough nerves in her spinal cord to paralyse her from the waist down. Removing the tumour could prevent the paralysis and keep her mobile for six to twelve months until the cancer grew back, and it could help with pain relief. The problem with this strategy was that any number of life-threatening complications could arise during the surgery, or in the two to three months in hospital after the operation.

'What kind of decision is that?' Pat snorted. 'The fact is, either way, I won't get in my kayak again. It sucks, right?' She looked at me sideways.

I nodded again. It did suck.

When I started out in the nursing profession in the 1980s, doctors often made these kinds of decisions for their patients. They recognised the burden on the sick person of making such a decision, and the stress on a family of second-guessing the decision after the fact. With the rightful decline in paternalism in medicine, and the increase in complexity of medical decisions, more and more patients are now faced with making such decisions, without sufficient knowledge or support to do so.

I glanced around the small suite that had been Pat's home for eight years. She'd moved there shortly after breaking up with her partner due to the stresses incurred by cancer. A cancer diagnosis often stretches a relationship beyond what it can withstand.

The big old television set kept her company through the long days when her friends were at work, along with stacks of CDs. Her favourite Saturday night activity had been to go dancing with friends. Framed photographs filled with ruddy outdoor faces from camping, hiking and kayaking trips adorned every available surface. In most of the photos Pat was in the centre, with friends on either side, her round face beaming with her mischievous smile. She called her huge circle of friends her 'chosen family'. The photographs filled the room with a vital past, unreachable in the future.

'I can't imagine not doing the surgery, that's the problem. To say no feels like curling up and waiting to die. Saying yes feels bold and courageous. I've become a symbol of hope for many of my cancer friends because I've lived so long with metastases. It sounds weird, but I can't let them down.' Pat blew her nose into a tissue.

'What if you don't have to be a hero any more? Maybe it's time to lay down your sword and say you can't fill that role any longer. It's too much pressure,' I said.

Pat's shoulders dropped an inch or two and she

sighed, looking down at the worn grey carpet beneath her old slippers.

'Perhaps your inspiration can take a different form now,' I continued. 'Maybe you can show your cancer friends what it looks like to surrender, that death doesn't have to be defied, or fought against, that there could be some grace in acceptance.'

Pat looked me in the eye. 'What a relief! I finally get to kick the bucket! I know I'm dying. I can pretend I'm not, or wish I wasn't, but if I'm honest with myself, whether I have this surgery or not, I'm done for.'

She picked up a box of Lindt chocolates and offered me one.

'I can eat as many chocolates as I want if I'm dying then, right?' she said. I popped one in my mouth and savoured the rush of sweetness.

'You always did anyway, no?' I responded.

'The surgery's such a huge unknown. I'd have to rely on my friends to visit me in hospital. They're all busy and I don't want to feel a burden.' Pat's brow was furrowed.

'What if they wanted to do that for you?' I said.

'Why would they? They'd rather be hiking.'

'Because they love you, maybe?'

'Oh yeah, they do love me. I suppose it's what you do, isn't it, when you love someone?'

Pat was exploring what surrender would feel like,

to die at home, cared for by her community. She'd seen many of her cancer friends die at home, or in hospice. Some had family and friends around them. Some didn't. Pat had more support than one person would ever need.

I felt the energy shift in the room before she spoke again.

'But I still can't think of *not* doing the surgery! The first thing I do when I wake up in the morning is try to move my legs. Waiting to become paralysed is torture. It's so scary.' Pat's voice became stronger.

'I have to try the operation. That's my nature. If given a challenge, I usually take it. You know that about me, Janie. Sitting here waiting to die, having people change my diapers and feed me, just doesn't do it for me.' Her will to act sparked again.

'I can't give up, Janie. I've got to try. You thought I was going to die four years ago, didn't you?' She liked her victory of having proved me wrong. 'I surprised you. Maybe I'll do it again!'

Four years earlier, everyone *did* think Pat was dying, including her oncologist. She weighed less than one hundred pounds and spent her days in and out of the palliative care unit for management of nausea and pain. To everyone's surprise, she bounced back and had four good years until the disease progressed again. I learned then not to fully trust a prognosis.

Pat continued. 'I just knew it wasn't my time. I don't know how you know these things, but you do. Like I know it will be my time soon but I'm just not sure how long it's going to take, that's all.'

The phone rang, piercing the intimacy.

'I'll call them back.' Pat was almost buoyant now, as though the strength of her decision finding its way up to the surface fuelled her energy.

Over and over again, Pat's determination had awed us. She had said yes to a hiking trip the summer before to Cathedral Lakes because she couldn't bear the idea of never seeing the Cascades again. She sent her five friends ahead of her on the trail because each step of hers would need breath she hardly had, and she worried she'd hold everyone up. Pat got herself to the top of Quiniscoe Mountain through sheer will and determination. She also got back in her kayak that summer and paddled around the Broken Islands one last time. Her eyes glistened when she told the story of paddling at sunset as whales passed nearby.

The decision about surgery was Pat's to make. People bring their whole lives, their personalities, their patterns, their fears and hopes to such life-and-death decisions. There is no right answer, just a thoroughly considered question.

I worried about the aftermath of surgery for Pat – the post-op pain, the potential for infection and other serious complications from being hospitalised for weeks on end. She might never get out. I had seen that happen countless times before, and sometimes I longed for the era before these aggressive surgeries when these types of decisions didn't have to be made at all.

'I have to try, Janie.' Pat's eyes blazed, her mind made up.

'I knew you'd figure this out. You always do.' My heart felt like it had collapsed in on itself and a wave of sorrow washed in behind my eyes. It was not up to me. 'Okay, so call the surgeon's office and find out if you are still booked for Thursday.'

'Thank God the decision is made,' she said. Pat looked older all of a sudden. We were both exhausted.

I stood up to leave, thinking the next time I would see Pat would be a few hours after surgery. I leaned over and gave her a hug.

'Call me and let me know if it's on for Thursday, and I'll see you at the end of the day.'

'Thanks again for coming by. You're the best but don't forget to have some fun, for goodness' sake.' Pat turned to lie down on the loveseat, lifting her legs up one at a time, using both arms. I tucked a cushion under her head. She'd be asleep in no time.

I let myself out the kitchen door, walked past the red, well-worn kayak hanging under the deck, and

into the bright October day. The buds on the helle-
bores that lined the small patch of grass in the front
garden had already formed. I hoped Pat would be
here in January to see them bloom.

'Janie,' the voicemail said at 5:32 on Wednesday
morning. 'I've changed my mind.'

'What happened?' I asked when I called Pat back.

'Life at any cost isn't worth it. I was wrestling most
of the night with my decision. I don't want to spend
the rest of my life in a hospital. I hate hospitals. And
what for? The cancer is going to get me in the end.
We all know that. Maybe being paralysed isn't the worst
thing. I have a friend in a wheelchair. He's not full
of self-pity. He just gets on with it. Being in hospital
dependent on pain pumps and nurses would be worse
than that,' Pat said. 'I can live well until I die. I think
I can even have fun. I've had four years I wasn't
supposed to have had. In fact, I've had eleven years I
wasn't expecting. When I had my first diagnosis, they
reckoned I'd have six months. I can't complain.' With
the torrent of words rushing out, she sounded excited.

'I love you, Pat,' I said. A rush of warm relief ran
through the centre of my body.

Two months after declining the surgery, Pat was weak
and confined to a wheelchair. Regardless, she was

determined to participate in the Christmas tradition with our Callanish staff and volunteers. It was 17 December and the plan was to meet at the Wedgewood Hotel in downtown Vancouver. The cosy lounge bar was beautifully festive with its plush red velvet couches, massive Christmas tree and twinkling white lights strung along the mantelpiece above the fireplace.

Pat's black cap was pulled down over her thinning grey-black hair, and her leather jacket hung loosely over black jeans. Her grin was as wide as ever, as she peered out of the back-seat window of the taxi.

'You made it! I'm so happy to see you,' I said.

'Well, what did you expect? A free Christmas cocktail at a place I could never afford to come to? Of course!'

Two of us leaned down and hoisted Pat out into the wheelchair. She could still stand, if she had someone to hold on to. She hadn't walked for the last three weeks.

'I'll have a mojito with an extra shot of rum, please,' Pat told the server. She didn't usually drink alcohol. 'And a mini pizza with caramelised onions and goat cheese.' She looked at us and smiled.

'What are you all looking so serious about? Lighten up, you guys. This is my last supper.'

We raised our glasses and Pat toasted.

'To good health.'

We all laughed.

'I do wonder sometimes if I should have done the surgery,' she said quietly, succumbing to a flash of regret. Death was close enough now to snuff out her spark for life and she could feel its presence.

Pat was admitted to a hospice two days later. Within another three days she was sleeping during the day for several hours at a time, no longer wanting or requiring food. In response to a familiar voice, she stirred from sleep to say a few words, a quip, like 'What are you all staring at?' or 'Haven't you got anything better to do?', and then she'd fall back asleep. The desire to connect with her friends, and the world around her, grew fainter in response to her waning energy. Even if she tried to fight it, she couldn't turn the tide. Pat had practised the art of surrender for many years. She had had to let go of most of what she loved in life, and accept the loss of her bodily functions, one at a time. Even the decision-making process itself set the stage for this ultimate surrender.

She died on 24 December 2010.

She had always hated Christmas.

9

GEORGE: Defying Death

George was too busy for cancer when he was first diagnosed. He was in his mid-forties, a high school teacher by day, and an involved father and husband on evenings and weekends. Colon cancer came out of the blue. He hadn't noticed anything unusual until the morning he saw drops of bright red blood in the toilet bowl. His wife Janet made the appointment for him to see their family doctor, insisting he make time to have the bleeding checked out.

George took the news of his cancer in his stride. He knew what he had to do and did it without much complaint. Bowel cancer was something he'd watched his father go through. Twenty-two years later, at seventy, his dad was as 'fit as a fiddle'. Twelve rounds of chemotherapy and six months after the diagnosis, George's cancer was in remission and life went pretty much back to normal, other than occasional jolts of fear on check-up days with the oncologist.

Three years later George was re-diagnosed with liver metastases secondary to the original diagnosis of colon cancer, and after the first few chemotherapies he had to be admitted to hospital for pain and symptom management, and a new regime of chemo-therapy. I was assigned to be his primary nurse, a fairly new role for me, having been at the BC Cancer Centre for just a year by then.

George and I talked about many things during the six weeks of his hospitalisation. He was a conscien-tious man and reminded me of my father, who after his own diagnosis of terminal cancer talked about wishing he had had more time in his life to develop his creative passions, like painting and writing poetry. By choice, both my father and George had made work and family life the priority. There had always been the assumption of time, later in life, for personal pursuits. George, like my father, wouldn't see his retirement years, and so those unrequited longings would remain unsettled in the heart, as many hopes of a lifetime often do.

The most illuminating conversations between patients and nurses often happen on night shifts, when the ward is quieter, and fears tend to surface with fewer distractions. One night, George told me that the chemotherapy wasn't working and that the oncologist that afternoon had offered him an experimental regime, one that would require several more weeks' stay in hospital. She would have to order it specially from the drug company on compassionate grounds, as it was unavailable to people like George who were not on a clinical trial. She expected the drug to take four or five days to arrive.

'I don't want to do it,' George said, in a quiet but resolute voice. 'Janet wants me to, but I know it won't do a thing. The time I have left is precious and I don't want to be stuck here in this hospital to see out the rest of my days.'

Many dying people slowly start to recognise that death cannot be defied, nor even kept at bay. Trying to prolong life, at the cost of dignity, made no sense to George. He wanted to live his last few months without a battle. Some family members accept the inevitability of the death of their loved ones, but some can't, and push hard to keep life going, to defy death. Giving up hope can be viewed as a withdrawal of love, a betrayal of the promise of for ever. Like in war, surrendering is not an option.

'It must be hard to be at odds with Janet about this,' I offered, not really knowing what to say.

Words often don't seem to help much in conversations such as the one George and I were having, and so I am grateful there are other ways nurses can offer care and comfort, such as with physical touch. I often remember the words of Florence Nightingale, 'I think one's feelings waste themselves in words; they ought all to be distilled into actions and into actions which bring results.'

'Would you like a back rub?' I asked. We often asked people if they wanted a back rub on the night shift, not something that happens much in hospitals nowadays. Nurses are assigned more patients than they can manage, and giving medications and doing computer work is often the mainstay of their work. They say there is not enough time to allow the pain to penetrate their busyness.

'Yes please, I'd like that. Janet is afraid to touch me these days, in case she hurts me. It's hard not to feel the touch of my sweetheart any more. You don't plan these things. One day the touching just stops.'

George rolled slowly onto his right side. Carefully pulling down the bedcovers to the edge of George's pyjama bottoms, I was grateful for the lineage of my profession, its long history offering such safe intimacy. George had already unbuttoned his pyjama top to make it easier for me to slip it over his shoulder.

I turned my attention to the lotion now warm in the palms of my hands. This back was unlike any other back I had rubbed lotion into. This back was showing me what death could look like. Gently, ever so gently, I moved my hands over the flaccid skin of his back, skin that had little muscle beneath to prop it up. My hands seemed to know what to do.

I ran the fingers of my right hand down the protruding bones of George's spine, my left hand massaging the soft muscles on either side. Each stroke wanted to communicate something. My hands wanted to tell George that whatever his body was doing, or not doing, he was still a whole person. The teacher, the father, the spouse, the feelings of accepting or giving up, feeling touchable or untouchable, all dissolved into the space between us. I wanted to say through my touch that at the end of a life, we still matter.

I heard George's breathing change. Each out-breath was longer than the one before; each seemed to embody a kind of letting go.

A small voice whispered, 'How do you say goodbye to your children when they still need you? Will Janet find them a new dad? I want that for her, even for them, and then I can't stand the thought of another man cheering them on at their games and taking them for ice cream on the way home.'

Unanswerable questions finding an unencumbered place to land.

I continued to stroke and gently knead the wasting

muscles of George's back. Even though I had no magic words with which to console his breaking heart, I felt strangely calm. Staying right where I was, listening with every fibre of my being, moving my hands gently, rhythmically, I instinctively knew it would help somehow.

George continued. 'I love my kids. I hope you get to meet them. Ben looks more like me, and Jess like her mom. I think they know I'm dying, but we haven't told them directly. I am not sure if we should, though I do think they have a right to know. Janet brings them here after school and I just tell them every day that I love them. I think they'll remember that. Ben says he is going to be a doctor when he grows up, so he can find a cure for cancer. Jess just wants me to tell her stories, like I did when she was young. Her favourites were always the ones I made up.'

The atmosphere in the room felt different all of a sudden. It was like an excruciating softness had fallen upon us. I felt a deep quiet inside, inexplicably at home in the presence of a man grappling with an unfathomable situation.

George closed his eyes. He had spoken all the words he was going to that night.

I had lost track of time. The faint light coming through the dirty hospital window was fading fast, although off in the distance I could see the bright lights of the helicopter pad announcing its location for the nighttime emergency arrivals from the north. I gently pulled up George's top sheet and the pale pink cotton blanket, leaving his arm free of his pyjama top so as not to wake him. I remember wishing hospitals had duvets, and soft feather pillows, and a vase of wildflowers in the corner. Placing the call bell within George's reach, I switched off his light, and thought better of planting a soft kiss on his cheek.

I had four days off following my conversation with George, and I thought about him and his decision as I went about my days. I hadn't yet learned to separate my work into a part of my brain that was inaccessible on my days off. The people I met lived inside me and I carried them around with me as I went about my life. It felt like I was keeping them company.

On my return to work, I was debriefed about the changes in George's condition, but even so, I was shocked when I entered his room on my first day back and saw how sick he had become in just four days. His skin had changed colour and was now a waxy, pallid shade of grey. Barely responsive, he looked like he was dying. I set about making George comfortable, with a slow gentle bed-bath and a change of pyjamas. I needed a second nurse to help me turn him in bed, as he could no longer move his own body at will. I combed his hair and shaved the previous day's growth off his chin with an electric razor. Janet would be in shortly and I wanted her to see how well cared for George was. His comfort might reassure her that dying could be bearable.

I felt her in the room before I saw her. The air crackled with anxiety as she entered. 'Will you be giving George his chemotherapy today?' Janet asked.

My heart sank. I had assumed that the decision to have chemotherapy was off the table now that George was dying.

'I didn't know he was having chemo today. Can we step out of the room for a moment and you can fill me in on what happened while I was off?' I didn't think this conversation should happen in front of George unless he could choose to participate.

We found an almost-quiet corner in the hallway between the nurses' station and the linen cupboard.

Janet rocked from one foot to the other as she spoke. 'We have to keep trying for the kids' sake. George is too young to die and he needs to keep fighting. The doctor has agreed that we should give it one more shot.'

'Did George make that decision?' I asked gingerly, knowing it was a risk.

'You can see he can't make his own decisions now. He would want me to make the decision for him.'

She looked at me accusingly, as though my questions were an affront to their marriage.

My stomach flipped. Being the primary care nurse, I would be assigned the task of giving George chemotherapy that day. As George's next-of-kin, Janet was now the substitute decision-maker.

I wish I'd had enough experience in those early days of my career to step towards Janet, to touch her arm, to look softly and directly into her eyes and ask her if she was frightened of what was happening to George, to her life. My young nurse's heart was pounding. I was afraid of her. Maybe the oncologist who prescribed the new chemotherapy was scared of her too, and didn't know how to tell her that more chemotherapy would be futile because her husband was dying.

I wanted to have the courage to say, *This is so hard, Janet, I am sorry this is happening. It's so sad for you and George, and the kids. None of it makes any sense. I wish it could be different but it can't be. George needs you to hear that he has had enough of fighting. He's not giving up; he just knows that he has come to the end of the road. He needs you to walk beside him for this part of the journey too, not just for the fighting part. I know you can do it. The kids need you to help them accept what is happening too.*

Perhaps Janet might have softened then, and collapsed into the relief of surrender. I didn't have the trust or courage to move towards Janet, though, rather than away.

The feeling of moral distress, a twisting and turning in the pit of my stomach, made me anxious. My jaw locked as the words that wanted to be spoken dried up in my mouth.

'I had a long conversation with George on Saturday night about treatment,' I attempted to explain. 'Can I tell you about it?' I asked.

'Sure, but it's wasting time, and every moment counts now. We have to blast those cancer cells, if he has any chance at all.' Janet looked over her shoulder towards the chemotherapy preparation room. Maybe she was hoping an IV bag with George's name on it would appear at any moment.

I felt the words I wanted to say float by me, lifted away by my fear and Janet's fear, all mixed up together.

I heard the clip-clip of her high heels on the hospital linoleum as she scurried away towards the nursing station, the sound of someone terrified to say goodbye.

My decision had begun to dawn on me from the inside out, like a secret illuminated by the act of truth-telling. I *had* to honour the conversation I had had with George a few days back. He had told me that he was tired, that the chance of an experimental chemo working was minuscule. He knew that death was close and accepted it was time to let go.

My heart thumped in my chest and my palms

sweated as I walked towards the head nurse's office. I needed to talk about this, even as temptation encircled me. I could carry on and give chemotherapy to George, like any other day. Why make such a fuss?

I had a good relationship with June, the head nurse. She was sitting at her desk when I entered the room.

'Do you have a minute? Can I close the door?' I asked.

'Of course, what's up?' She spun around in her chair to look me in the eye. June was one of those head nurses who transmitted confidence. No matter the crisis, she knew what to do. Her short white hair gelled into spikes seemed to emphasise her competence.

'George is slated to have chemotherapy today. I don't think he should be getting it.' I thought I might as well get to the point.

'Why's that?' June looked at me with concern.

'George told me on Saturday night that he's done with treatment. He's had enough. He knows he's dying. Today he's barely conscious and definitely not competent to make this decision himself now. Janet must have made the decision for him, and of course she wants to hold on to the last vestiges of hope.' The tension of holding back tears burned in my throat.

'Have you talked to Janet about your concerns?' June asked.

'I tried, but I didn't get very far. She feels it's her

decision to make now.' I could feel my tears being replaced by anger.

'It *is* Janet's decision to make, Janie,' she said gently.

I felt George's autonomy slipping away, and my own courage. I found myself searching for the torn pieces of an ancient cloth that has always wrapped life and death together as one. Accepting our loved ones will die opens us to life's impermanence, to our aloneness. Fighting to the very end can separate us from them too soon and prevents the potential for a solid goodbye. I knew Janet was inside a prison and that neither my skill, nor the system itself, could help her take down the walls.

My anger receded as I acknowledged that June was right. As his wife, she could make the decision for George, one that I could not support. In place of the anger was the comfort of a steady resolve. I knew what I had to do.

'June, I can't do it.' My voice was soft but non-negotiable.

June glanced at me sideways. 'What do you mean?'

'I have to honour the conversation I had with George. He didn't want more chemotherapy. I won't be the one giving it to him today.'

'Ask Mary to give George the chemo and then why don't you go home? You look tired. We'll talk about this tomorrow,' she said, weariness infusing her voice.

I turned to go. 'Thanks, I will,' I said.

Walking past George's open door, I paused to see if Janet was anywhere to be seen.

'She went to get a coffee,' the unit clerk said. She'd likely overheard the conversation Janet and I had had in the corner of the hallway. Her smile assured me I had an ally.

Moving quickly, I approached the bed. George smelled like death, the familiar rancid odour of decay. His breathing was loud and I could hear the crackle of secretions in the back of his throat, his cough reflex too weak to clear them. I knew that even though he was sleeping, hearing is the last sense to fade and that he'd very likely be aware of everything that was said in his presence.

'George. Take good care,' I whispered. The words were wrong and lacked the courage of a direct farewell. 'I just want you to know I heard what you said the other night about not wanting more treatment. Janet is scared of being in the world without you, of course, so she wants to keep fighting on your behalf. Nurse Mary will give you the chemo today. You are doing this for Janet, and perhaps that is okay with you. I can't give it to you because I know it's not what you want.' I brushed his cheek with the back of my hand. George stirred ever so slightly.

'Bye, George,' I whispered and slipped out of the

room without looking back. Emerging into the bright sunlight on the street, I felt the gentle brush of my destiny pass by. I recognised that a different kind of medicine was calling me home.

III.

HEALING THE TROUBLED HEART

*'Pain is important: how we evade it, how we succumb to it,
how we deal with it, how we transcend it.'*

—AUDRE LORDE

For many people, in order to come to terms with dying there is work they wish to do: to grieve the unattended sorrows of a lifetime; to rage against past hurts; to try to forgive oneself or others or, at least, to accept what has happened; to settle fears and worries; to say goodbye to family and friends; and to leave a legacy.

Choosing to open our hearts to dying requires that we feel the many emotions that will undoubtedly arise, such as sadness, regret, anger, disappointment, self-blame, guilt, envy, love, peace and many others. To have the courage to open our hearts to our feelings offers us the possibility for deep healing before we die. Revealing our pain to a group of witnesses willing to hear our suffering without judgement can carry us out of isolation and into a community that offers a sense of belonging.

I have been deeply moved by the work I have seen people do to free themselves before they die, or to take care of their closest people after they are gone. I have seen how the pain instilled by early loss has become the catalyst for choosing a meaningful life which becomes the healing.

I met Naomi for the first time when she was thirteen. Her enormous blue eyes took me in as we shook hands at the door. She had retreated safely behind those eyes somewhere, which wasn't surprising given her mom was dying of ovarian cancer.

The family meeting had been arranged by Naomi's mother Tamar, who wanted to talk with her three children and her husband about what lay ahead for her, and for them. I feel it is an act of great love and courage when a dying person takes care of their family in this way. Many people understandably shy away from these excruciating conversations. Naomi was quiet throughout the meeting, present and absent at the same time. Her two older siblings, her dad and her mom talked and cried, and talked some more. They were preparing.

The second time Naomi and I met was ten years later, after she had phoned me out of the blue.

'Hi Janie, I don't know if you remember me?' she said, her voice bright and warm.

'Of course I remember you,' I said. I had heard a few stories about her from her dad and her brother and sister, whom I continued to see from time to time, but had often wondered how Naomi had fared after her mom died.

'I'm in first-year medical school at UBC,' she said. 'I have a six-week flex course which I can design myself, and I wonder if I can spend time with you to learn about the non-medical ways to help families living with cancer. They won't teach me those things at medical school.' Her words tumbled out with excitement. She had found her voice now, at twenty-three, and I could hear the self-confidence in her voice.

'Of course, I would love to have you here at Callanish,' I said, my eyes filling with surprised tears. I could feel her mom's pride for her daughter ripple through the air to meet mine.

Naomi told me that when her mom was very sick, she used to leave home every evening by herself and walk and cry, and walk and cry, and she always wondered why no one ever stopped a thirteen-year-old girl out at night by herself, crying, to ask if she was okay. Until one day, an elderly man with a kind voice asked, 'Is everything all right, dear?' Naomi told the man she was okay, even though she wasn't, because she couldn't talk about her mom to anyone then, especially not to a stranger. In that moment of connection with the man she described feeling waves of gratitude flood through her, for being cared about by someone who didn't need to know her story to offer her a moment of kindness.

Naomi told me that her mom had recorded audio tapes and written an ethical will for each of the three kids to have after she died, and that her mom's wisdom had guided her in every challenging decision she had made in her life so far.

Her mom wrote in her journal: *My legacy of who I was as a person will give them guidance in life and facilitate kindness, goodness and love that will embrace them in their journey through life.*

Naomi spent six weeks at Callanish talking to parents about the importance of leaving legacies for their children. The legacy work her mother had done has helped many other parents and their children.

The four stories in *Healing the Troubled Heart* describe the courage and strength it takes for people to do the emotional and spiritual work that can liberate them before they die, and for the legacies they leave for their families and the world.

10

BELLA: Soul Retrieval

'I have a hole in my soul,' Bella said when I asked her why she had come on retreat. 'It's been that way for as long as I can remember.'

It was a cool and sunny November afternoon when Bella pulled up into the parking lot of the retreat centre. I noticed a whiff of cigarette smoke as I lugged her suitcase out of the trunk of her SUV, while she gathered up several smaller bags from the back seat. Metastatic cancer likely made quitting smoking pointless. Her black coat reached almost to the ankles of her fur-lined winter boots and her silver hoop earrings hung to her collar.

'You never know what you might need,' she laughed apologetically at the overladen luggage cart. 'Never been to something like this before; not sure if it's my thing.'

I imagined it must have taken a lot of courage for Bella to step out of her comfort zone and come on a retreat, not knowing any of the other group participants or the staff, and having not been on a retreat before. I often wonder if some people, like Bella, come in response to a call from a deeper part of themselves – their soul, one might say – when it is in need of healing. It often only makes sense to them after the retreat is over.

We lingered on the wide footbridge that spanned Brew Creek, the water high and fast-flowing after the autumn rains.

'It's nice here,' she said. 'Maybe it'll be okay after all?' She looked at me sideways.

I nodded. 'I think it will.'

We sat side-by-side on the queen-sized bed in one of six guest rooms upstairs in the main lodge. Bella's eyes settled briefly on the vase of dusky pink lilies and white gerberas on the bedside table, and the hand-made card that said *Welcome to the Callanish Retreat* tucked in between one of the puffy pillows and the down comforter.

'This folder contains the schedule for the week and information about your group and our facilitator team,' I said, opening the navy folder that had *BELLA* typed on its cover.

'Sure,' she whispered, as she took off her glasses.

She was crying. 'It's such a relief to be here after all I've been through. Life's hard when you live alone, with no one to bring you a cup of tea, or to tell you to buck up. It's just me and my kitty and I get lonely.' She reached for a tissue from the box on her bedside table and wiped her eyes.

After a few moments, Bella composed herself and then continued. 'Last month, when my oncologist told me the breast cancer had spread to my liver, my first thought was, *I'm going to die without ever having really lived*. Dying doesn't scare me, but my life being a complete sham does. I've given myself a week to figure out this living business. Do you think I can do it?'

'Well, let's give it a good try,' I said, touching her shoulder as though to seal the intention.

I stood to go, leaving her to unpack. 'See you downstairs for our introductory circle at five-thirty, okay?' I said. Bella had already begun the process of healing.

The muffled voice of another team member welcoming a participant drifted down the hallway, and the smell of onions and garlic announced that dinner was under way. Other newcomers were settling into a five-bedroom house a few minutes' walk down the wooden pathway, across from the creek and the hot tub. An hour or so after arrival the group gathered in the lounge for the welcome session to go over the programme schedule, logistics and staff introductions before dinner.

The dining room was quiet for the first meal of the retreat, with only an occasional murmur between two people attempting to find common ground. I looked forward to the buzz of chatter and laughter in the room that would accompany the last meal, once people had got to know one another and laid down their burdens.

After dinner, the participants shared their stories about cancer. They were invited to speak for as long as they wished, and could start anywhere along the trajectory of illness. They were encouraged to listen to one another without verbally responding, reacting or interrupting and, when one person finished, to pause before the next person shared. Being able to articulate a story in the quiet embrace of a silent circle ensures that the speaker, no matter how vulnerable, feels a strong sense of safety. And within that space, words can be spoken freely and healing can begin.

The fire crackled in the river-rock hearth and the wind pushed itself up against the windowpanes. A smattering of snow covered the ground outside, although winter had not yet fully set in.

One person at a time spoke of how it felt to hear the words 'You have cancer.' They described the rigours of surgery, chemotherapy and radiation, and shared feelings of fear, anger, sadness and uncertainty. Former lives were shattered, their new lives unrecognisable. They hoped to find ways to grieve their losses, deal with their anger, and learn to live with uncertainty so they could find joy again.

Some of the stories tumbled out, words falling over each other, eager to land in the warmth of caring attention. Details that had been stored away in memory were coaxed out by the honesty of others. Some stories were spare and searing. Life would be cut short by a recurrence of cancer and future plans dissolved into an ending that was closer than expected. Children would become parentless, and grandchildren not yet born would never be known.

Others revealed enquiring minds, asking unanswerable questions: *Why me? Why now? How long?* They grappled to make sense of a life that wasn't supposed to unfold this way. A burst of inconsolable weeping was allowed to run its course or silence was held while the group waited for the speaker to continue.

Then came a rush of welcome laughter as Bella confessed to the group that she had driven her own vehicle to the retreat, rather than accept the ride offered, in case she needed to escape.

On the third morning the conversation turned to mothers and fathers. This particular group of eight had much in common in terms of their difficult childhoods. Each person described the parents who raised them with stories of neglect and abuse, alcoholism and suicide. They spoke of themselves as children who were scared, lonely, rebellious and alienated, with childhoods they wished to forget. They wanted to put their painful memories to rest so they could live whatever time they had left unburdened by the past.

Bella had had a very rough start in life. Her father had taken his own life when she was nine years old. She remembers waking up and being told by her mother that her dad had died unexpectedly in the night. No one spoke of it again. Two years after his death, Bella's mother married John, an abusive man. At eleven, Bella had no choice but to live with her mom and new stepfather.

As traumatic memories began to surface, Bella chose her next words carefully. 'I can't talk about that kind of evil, here in this beautiful room, with all of you. He isn't worthy of our attention.' Her lips set into a thin hard line, as though to prevent any more syllables from pushing their way out of her mouth, contaminating the atmosphere.

The break for lunch was welcome after a dive into the shadows of the past. The trees that lined the creek path steadied us as the retreat group and facilitators ambled back towards the lodge. Breathing in the edge of winter on the cold mountain wind brought us back to the present time.

The borscht and fresh soda bread was set out on the lunch table, with spinach salad topped with dried cranberries and pumpkin seeds. Bella didn't seem to have much of an appetite, pushing the spinach leaves around on her plate.

A small log cabin on the property, converted into an art studio for the retreat, straddled the creek – its continuous gurgle audible from inside the room. One of the large windows framed the bare branches and white bark of the aspen grove, and from the opposite window the creek stretched towards the bridge bordered by snowberry bushes.

Nature plays a vital part in the healing process, inviting a shift in awareness from an intensely personal experience to a shared, even universal, reality. Orienting to a larger view can help one feel less alone and more connected to the world.

At dusk, the group gathered around the art table accompanied by Gretchen, the retreat art therapist, and two other facilitators. Two chunks of clay lay on a square of cardboard in front of each participant; one piece could fit easily into the palm of a hand.

Gretchen's voice was soft and encouraging. 'You

might wish to close your eyes and place the palms of your hands on top of the clay. Notice the coolness of these little pieces of earth in your hands. For centuries, people around the world have put their hands on clay to design and decorate objects or symbols to use, to play with, to wear, or to worship. We will use the clay this afternoon to help us gain insight about the complex relationships we have with our parents.'

One of the essential skills of an art therapist is to put people at ease. Many people were discouraged from being creative when they were young, or shamed into believing they had no artistic abilities.

'Don't think of making anything specific, just let your hands do what they instinctively want to do with the clay.' Around the table people had begun to push or roll, mould or sculpt the clay as if something, or someone, was telling them what to do. Some kept their eyes closed; others opened their eyes and were intensely focused on the clay. Hands moved and shapes began to appear.

Bella pushed one of her two pieces of clay out of reach and slowly began to roll the other on the table with her right hand, back and forth, over and over, shaping it into a cylinder about six inches long, a frown line between her eyebrows deepening while she worked.

One woman formed a pile of tiny clay balls the size of marbles, rolling each one carefully between the palms of her hands. Another smoothed out a flat heart the size of a hand, rhythmically stroking the surface with the pads of two fingers. Quiet piano notes floated through the room, played by Maryliz, our retreat musician; the lilt of the improvised melody mirrored the mood and helped sustain people's focus.

Bella stood up urgently and walked over to the side table that was covered with art supplies: paints, fabrics and paper. She rummaged through a pile of material scraps, then took a pair of scissors and cut some coarse brown fabric into an eight-inch square. A smile came over her face as she began to wrap the sackcloth around the cylinder of clay.

'Just so I don't have to touch him with my bare hands,' she whispered to me. Bella cut several feet of twine from the roll and wound it around the fabric-covered clay, from top to bottom. Her twisting gained vigour, wrapping around and around until she had about three feet of twine left dangling towards the floor. Abruptly, she shoved the piece away from her towards the centre of the table. She averted her gaze from the clay to the water-soaked paper towel she was using to clean her hands. She was finished for now.

Once everyone stopped working, Gretchen asked people to speak about their experience, if they wished to. When it came to Bella's turn, she said she wasn't ready to talk. Everyone nodded, respectful of her privacy, and when they left the room for dinner Bella stayed behind.

'It's him! He's here, and now I have to do something with him. It might have to be rather horrible,' she said, looking at Gretchen and me with a vengeful air. The man who had abused her for years was now under her control for the first time in her life.

'Let us know if you need our help with what comes next,' Gretchen said. She touched Bella lightly on her shoulder. 'Take your time to think about it. Maybe it will be revealed in your dreams tonight?'

Bella nodded. 'He will have to wait at least until I've had dinner, and probably until I've had a good night's sleep. I'll shove him in this dark corner under the table, to ponder his fate.' Her voice was clear. She was in charge now.

The next morning Bella asked her retreat friends if they would witness the disposal of a negative force in her life. She needed to retrieve a piece of her soul that had been taken over by darkness, and she asked if the group would accompany her on the forest path to find the right spot for the disposal. Donning boots, scarves and winter jackets, the group set out with Bella along the creekside path towards the rainforest. Bella hadn't wanted to put on boots, and her painted toenails in gold flip-flops seemed to spit in the face of winter.

The sackcloth object dangled almost to the ground by Bella's side, one end of the brown twine held tightly in her right glove, and in the other hand she carried a shovel. After about a ten-minute walk, Bella stopped and looked into the forest to the left of the path. 'This marsh looks perfect,' she announced. The dank earth was dotted with skunk cabbage.

'I've wanted to bury this asshole since the moment I met him. He was buried after he died, but I didn't go to his funeral. So now I'm going to free myself from this dark force, with your help. But first, I'm going to drag him through the scum!' Bella marched over to a stagnant puddle of black water and slowly lowered the clay piece into the darkness. Then she dragged it back and forth several times before yanking it out. She was enjoying herself now.

'Okay, you're going down, once and for all.' She shoved him aside as she began to dig a hole in the dark earth. I was surprised at her stamina for the job. When the hole was a foot or so deep, and she was panting, she said, 'Forget it, you don't deserve to take up any more of our precious time.' She was speaking directly to the object lying off to the side of the hole.

Bella picked up the end of the string and tossed the figure into the opening with indifference. She quickly pushed a pile of soil over the hole with the shovel, without looking in.

'Now for the finale.' She glanced up at the group of twelve witnesses standing at the edge of the path, dropped the shovel, and with both feet jumped a few inches in the air before landing hard down on to the newly covered pit, her golden flip-flops sinking into the dark loam.

'Good riddance.' She brushed her hands back and forth a few times and turned to face her new friends. Expressions of relief covered tear-stained faces.

'My soul says thank you,' she said.

Six months later, Bella told me that the hole in her soul had filled in. She couldn't trust it completely, but she had started to imagine a brighter life, for however long it lasted. Almost two years after the retreat, Bella chose to spend her last weeks at a hospice not far from her home. Her sister brought her cat in to visit whenever she could. She responded to my knock on the door of her private room with a hearty, 'Come in if you dare. I don't bite.' I sensed that this might be my last visit with Bella.

No hospital gowns for her; she wore an ankle-length black, teal and crimson nightgown with a matching teal cardigan, and her lips were glossy with balm. Her hair had thinned from the latest and final round of chemotherapy, and her translucent pallor showed a bloodstream deprived of haemoglobin. Bella asked if we could walk outside for our visit, a last-ditch effort for independence, and for what would likely be one of her last puffs on a cigarette.

'Will you let me take your arm?' I asked.

'All right, if it makes you feel better.' I could feel the soft skin of her underarm hang from its bone without muscle to hold it in place. We ambled past mostly closed doors to the atrium, with its cosy lounge for families to sit and pass the time. I pushed open the heavy front door and felt the welcome waft of fresh air. Bella wanted to show me the garden, with its late summer asters and black-eyed Susans in the perennial border around a square of well-tended grass. She hadn't been well enough to tend her own garden that summer.

The September sunshine was low in the sky but it was warm enough to sit on a wooden bench tucked under a Japanese maple. Bella asked for updates about her retreat friends, and the staff team, and I gave her the news. She hadn't lost her interest in the people she cared about and I relaxed into what felt like a conversation that we would continue to have long after she was gone.

'Are you settled in yourself?' I asked. 'Ready for the unknown?'

'I am, Janie. I'm ready to go. All my soul-searching has paid off. My unfinished business is done, enough at least for one life. My soul is ready for its next journey.' Bella reached for my hand.

'How do you think the hole in your soul got mended?' I asked.

'Well, how do you think?' Bella laughed.

'I think your hard work on retreat paid off,' I said.

Bella nodded. 'I feel like I retrieved the parts of myself that went missing long ago, thanks to all of you, and the hole filled in. I wish I'd known how to do that years ago, but at least it happened before I died holey,' she chuckled, as she stubbed her cigarette butt out with the toe of her black suede ballerina slipper. She then slowly reached down to pick it up. 'Still pretending to everyone else I'm not smoking,' she said, as she poked the stub into her cardigan pocket.

I noticed a rush of warmth fill my chest, which I understood to be deep gratitude and a sense of completion in our relationship. Our work together was done and I felt hopeful – hopeful for all the people who believe they cannot come to peace with a horror that has become part of the fabric of their being. Bella had shown me that it was possible to be free.

II

ANNELIESE: Released

Anneliese wasn't sure why she'd grabbed the small glass bottle of soil off her dresser minutes before she left for the retreat. On her most recent visit to Würzburg, she had gathered a handful of soil from her mother's grave to take home. Her mother died in 1971, at the age of thirty-four, when Anneliese was six years old.

'After a while the grave gets used for someone else,' she told me. 'Another body goes in on top, unless you keep paying for the lease. I'm not sure my mom would have liked a stranger, some Karl Schmidt, being thrown in on top of her.' She paused. 'But then again, knowing Mom, she might have?' Anneliese's throaty chuckle was infectious.

The rain held off under thin grey November clouds and a sliver of blue had opened up in the distance over Black Tusk mountain. Anneliese's fellow retreat participants gathered on the grass beside a wide curve of the creek to witness a funeral that Anneliese hadn't been allowed to attend forty-three years earlier. Anneliese was looking her own death squarely in the face. She had metastatic breast cancer, the same disease that her mom had died from.

I looked around the circle of retreat participants and staff members who mingled on the creekside on that cool winter morning, willing to support Anneliese to close a chapter of her life. I always feel hopeful when I witness how relative strangers have a natural willingness to support healing in others. Perhaps we can't heal ourselves on our own and it is our very interdependence that is the essential medicine for healing.

On the first day of the retreat, she had whizzed into the parking lot in an ancient Pontiac Sunrunner emitting blue smoke from its muffler. The front passenger seat had been removed to make space for her companions in life: Murphy, her thirteen-year-old Lab, and Edie, her Lab/pit bull cross. Her biggest concern before the retreat had been to find someone to mind her dogs and her thoroughbred horse, Mexxy, for a whole week. Anneliese tugged her red knitted toque down over her ears as she hopped out of the car. Not having hair in winter was bitter.

'That was quite the journey!' she said. 'Nine hours' drive! My oncologist told me I should come on retreat, and I trust her, so here I am! By the way, call me Ahnna-Leece. It's the German way.'

I wheeled her well-worn suitcase across the wooden bridge, pointing out the hot tub to the right of us, and the art cabin on our left.

We had used the Brew Creek Centre every season for twelve years by then, a mountain lodge set in the midst of twelve acres of old-growth Douglas firs, large-leaf maples and cedars, on land that has been the traditional territory of the Squamish and Lil'Wat First Nations since time immemorial. Maureen, our Cree friend, who joins our staff team from time to time, feels the presence of the ancestors on the land there and says prayers each night to thank them for their presence, and to ask them for help with the healing work that happens on retreat.

The crackle of the fire greeted Anneliese and me as we entered the front door of the lodge.

'Welcome to Callanish and to your home for a week,' I said.

One corner of Anneliese's mouth turned up into a wry smile. 'Someone told me this retreat is hard work. Was that you?'

'Probably,' I said. 'It will be worth it, I promise you.' After facilitating sixty-eight weeklong retreats by then, I had some confidence in the process.

After dinner, Anneliese was the first of eight retreatants to tell her story to the eighteen people who sat in armchairs around the fireplace in the lounge. The staff of ten included the retreat facilitators and the kitchen team, who all joined the circle every evening.

Anneliese cut to the chase. 'I'm not ready to die. Forty-nine is too young. I've got fifteen years on my mom, who died of the same cancer as me, but it's the anger I have to deal with. I've been angry since the day my oma told me Mom died, and then forbade me from crying.' Anneliese looked into the faces of strangers.

As I listened to her, I pondered how we often shelve difficult experiences for later, but the past wants to be settled, like the unfinished books we abandon that call to us as we pass by the bookshelf. Perhaps putting things off fuels the illusion we might live for ever.

Anneliese emigrated to Canada in her mid-twenties and worked as a nanny until she received her permanent residency status and went to university to study psychology.

'I moved to Kamloops for a good job but had to leave when my cancer came back. I had such high hopes for my career. Everything changes after cancer, and that's difficult to accept.' Anneliese's eyes glanced around the circle, like a child seeking reassurance from new friends.

The story tumbled out of her. 'After Mom died, my aunt moved in to help my dad, and they hated each other. I felt like the leftover kid; my dad favoured my older brother and my aunt preferred my younger brother,' she told the group, as memories came to find her.

'I didn't expect to talk about all this here, but it feels good. Thanks for listening,' she said, rushing back into present time. Her large hands gripped each other as though they were telling her she'd said enough, that she had taken up too much space.

The following afternoon, in an unoccupied bedroom upstairs in the lodge, Anneliese sat cross-legged on the bed with her back pushed into a couple of pillows, and I perched on a wooden desk chair with my feet propped up against the boxspring.

The winter sun had set at four-thirty p.m. and through the window behind where Anneliese sat dusk was waiting for the arrival of night.

I leaned in. 'I like to meet with each person for an hour or so during the retreat, so if there's anything you'd like to talk about, this is a good time,' I said.

Anneliese's smile was tentative. 'What should I do with all this anger? It's killing me,' she said. 'Literally.'

'What does the anger feel like in your body?' I asked.

'It's like a huge pressure on my chest on the verge of exploding.'

'Have you ever exploded?'

'No, I just keep moving. I never sit still. I think I'm scared to stop.' Her piercing blue eyes fixed my gaze.

'Fear and sorrow are often buried under anger,' I said. 'What might you be afraid of?'

'I've been scared for as long as I can remember, terrified of the zombies, the walking dead who threatened to kill me in the night. That's why I never slept as a kid. The zombies still scare me.'

I reached for what lay beneath the fear. 'Tell me about your mom.'

'She was gorgeous. Everyone said so. She was tall like me and had shiny dark hair swept up off her forehead like they did in the forties, dark eyes and a regal nose, like mine.' She turned her head to show me her profile. 'She was full of laughter and was loved by everyone who knew her. I know she adored us.' Anneliese's face lit up in the remembering.

'You sound like you are describing yourself, minus the hair of course,' I said, assuming she could take the quip.

'I think I am like her,' she smiled. 'Why would a family send a kid away when their mom is sick? I felt like I was being punished.' Anneliese looked up at me, expecting a response to this new information.

'Perhaps they were trying to protect you rather than punish you?'

'From what?'

'From seeing your mom in so much pain.'

'Maybe, but my brothers got to stay. Why didn't they need protecting? It has always felt like they hated me,' she said. 'Even when I came home after she died, it felt like that.'

Her face communicated the shock that was inflicted long ago. A freezing effect registered in her facial muscles, in the skin stretched taut across cheekbones, and in the flatness of eyes that had witnessed too much.

'I am so sorry your mom died,' I said. 'She has missed so much, seeing who you are today, knowing what you have accomplished in your life.'

Anneliese's pencilled-in eyebrows lifted in surprise. 'No one has ever said that to me. The nuns in kindergarten told me that I was the devil-spawn, that it was my fault she was sick, and because of me she'd die.'

Stories of childhood abuse shock me with their cruelty no matter how many times I hear them. One of the challenges for any therapist or counsellor is not to become immune to the stories, but to hear them as though for the first time. We also must not ask too many questions about the stories, in an attempt to understand how these horrible things can happen. These questions can convey doubt that shuts a person's feelings down.

In this case, an immediate response rushed out of me. 'That's terrible; that should never have been said to you. You were just a little girl. No wonder you felt like everyone hated you.'

Guilt was wedged inside Anneliese. She felt responsible for her mother's death, and only one person could release her from it. 'Would it be okay to imagine your mom is here with us?' I asked.

'I'd like that,' she said.

'Sometimes we don't think to talk to a person who has died. Can you imagine what she might want to say to you, if she was here today?'

Anneliese paused for several moments, waiting for her mother's voice.

'*Es war nicht deine Schuld, meine Liebe. Niemand verursachte meinen Tod. Es war Krebs, der mich von dir wegnahm. Ich hätte alles getan, um zu bleiben und deine Mutter zu sein. Alles.*' An exquisite tenderness emanated from the words of Anneliese's first language.

'In English now,' she said, 'for you to understand.'

'*It wasn't your fault, my love. No one caused my death. It was cancer that took me away from you. I would have done anything to stay and be your mom. Anything.'* A tear hung suspended on the end of Anneliese's nose for a few seconds before she reached for a tissue.

Giving her some privacy, I glanced out of the window. The fragments of sky between the branches of the aspens had turned indigo, an impossible colour to replicate on a paint palette.

When our eyes reconnected, Anneliese spoke:

'I've needed to hear those words from my mom all these years, to know that it wasn't my fault. I really believed those nuns. Thank you for helping me.'

'Your body remembers your mom's love. Without the anger and guilt, you'll be able to feel that love more easily,' I said.

Anneliese nodded. 'I hope so. That would be nice. But there's one more thing, Janie, that's always bothered me,' she said. 'I wish I'd been allowed to go to her funeral. My dad didn't think I could handle it, but I could have, you know? That's probably why I haven't been able to let her go.'

'Would you like to have a funeral here at Brew Creek for her?' I asked. 'You didn't get to say goodbye.' It's never too late to pay respects to the people we love.

'I'd like that,' Anneliese said. 'You know, some part of me must have known I'd be doing this when I grabbed the soil on my way out the front door. I will give Mom her final resting place here at Brew Creek.'

In the group art session the next morning, Anneliese fashioned a small bowl out of pottery clay. She then sculpted a cupped right hand, carefully delineating each finger and fingernail so that it could cradle the bowl. She asked Gretchen, our art therapist, to mould a left hand to match the right, perhaps evoking the company of her mom through Gretchen's presence. Both hands were then joined together and the small clay bowl was placed inside the hands. She unscrewed the lid of the glass bottle and shook the soil into the clay bowl. The urn was ready for its resting place.

'I can't do this yet,' Anneliese announced to the group. 'I've got to do something with my anger first. That feeling like I'm about to explode is back. All those nights alone as a kid, afraid of the zombies. It was horrible.' Anneliese had broken into a sweat and her chest was heaving.

'Why don't we take a walk outside?' I asked her.

'Good idea, maybe stomping around in the forest will help,' she said.

We walked up the creek path to a dense grove of Western red cedars. The earth was spongy underfoot when we veered off the trail. Stepping over fallen branches and around nurse logs, Anneliese led us deeper into the darkness of the rainforest. She seemed to know where she was going.

'Aha!' she said. 'Now we're getting there. Needs to be really private. Even living in my small town in the boonies, you can't let go of anger. You'd scare your neighbours and they'd call the police.'

With one hand braced against the bark of an old-growth cedar, Anneliese let out a blood-curdling scream. 'I hate you, death!' she shrieked into the darkness. 'I hate you.' Falling to her knees then, she collapsed into sobs on the damp forest floor. I moved closer, my right hand touching the strength of the tree beside me.

Anneliese's body shuddered as each wracking sob crashed through. Gradually the sobs became whimpers, and after a few moments she turned her head, my signal to speak.

'May I put my hand on your back?' I asked, kneeling down beside her.

'Sure,' she said.

I laid the palm of my hand between her shoulder blades and slowly rubbed in wide circles over her upper back for comfort. The swathes of cedar boughs above our heads in their own wide circle offered a magnanimous surround.

'Perhaps we should get back to the group. They might be worried about us,' she said after a few minutes, perking up.

'Are you ready to go back?' I asked.

'That scream was fifty years overdue. I'm more than ready. Plus, I'm famished.'

Anneliese stood up, brushed the brown splinters of cedar off her damp knees, and set off for the lodge, her hunger a sure sign that she had laboured hard.

Anneliese invited her retreat friends to come to the funeral the following day. Some of them also bore unattended sorrows, and grieved alongside her. She cradled the clay hands with her own as she strolled down the footpath from the art studio to the grass where the group had gathered. It was as though the red willow stems and the bare paper-bark maples along the creekside witnessed her as she passed by. Even the sun embraced her with its generous winter light.

Heads bowed low as eyes rested inside the bowl that Anneliese showed each person around the circle, one at a time.

'Thank you for being here with me today,' she said. 'It is amazing that I can do this, after all these years.'

I followed Anneliese as she clambered down the shallow bank to the tiny rocky beach. She turned to face her retreat friends on the grass above. Her cheeks glistened with tears, though she beamed a wide smile.

'I have held on to Mom for more than forty years

because I didn't know how to say goodbye. Letting her go today means I can finally be at peace.'

Anneliese waded into the centre of the rushing creek in the rubber boots she had borrowed from a retreat friend. The edges of her long coat dipped into the icy water as she bent low to place the clay bowl into the water, settling it on top of smooth, round rocks.

'Wow! Did you see that?' She looked up at me with a grin.

'No,' I said. 'What happened?'

'As soon as I put the bowl down, the water whooshed the soil out, lickety-split. I guess she was ready to go?'

The sound of a flute rippled above our heads, the high notes seeming to lift us into a space where death and life abide together. I looked over and saw Maryliz tucked in between two trees on the opposite riverbank, her silver flute glinting in the sun. Anneliese took my arm in hers as we stood quietly in the pale winter sunshine and watched the water caress the clay bowl sitting in its midst. The bowl would take a few hours to dissolve, the clay fingers holding on until they, too, could release their hold.

I offered Anneliese a small glass bowl filled with rose petals – red, orange and white – gathered from posies brought from each participant's bedside, the rich velvet blooms offering beauty into the heartbreak of cancer.

She scooped up a handful and tossed them into the water. The colours danced on the sparkling current as they eddied downstream, eliciting a collective gasp from the onlookers. Each person, one at a time, stepped off the bank to the creek's edge and threw a handful of petals into the rushing water as the clouds scurried overhead in the cold breeze as though they also had somewhere to go.

Anneliese was greeted with congratulatory hugs as she scrambled back up onto the grass.

'That was amazing. Good for you,' those gathered cried.

'Can I play the song now?' Anneliese asked me, her voice buoyant, pointing to the wireless speaker she had set on the picnic table close by. 'My mom gave me the single "Wild Thing" before she died and I've played it thousands of times and I want to share it with all of you.'

The Troggs boomed out and the bass thumped under the vocals.

Anneliese grabbed my right hand, and Gretchen's left hand, and lifted our arms high over our heads. She swayed her body back and forth as though there was no cancer living in her liver or bones. Every person had taken hands in theirs and was rocking and singing too.

Anneliese's voice could be heard over all the others.

The final conversation I had with Anneliese was at the hospice, five months after the retreat. One of her friends had brought in her dogs, Murphy and Edie, for a visit the day before. Anneliese told me how much she missed them and how she loved having them jump up on her bed and lick every inch of her face, swollen from the effects of steroids.

Although bedbound due to extensive swelling in her legs, Anneliese was cheerful. 'You'll think I'm crazy, Janie, but I still think I'm going to get better,' she said. Hope has a way of infusing a strong spirit, even when the body is failing.

Anneliese died three weeks later, just twelve weeks short of her fiftieth birthday.

12

KIRSTEN: Writing on Purpose

Kirsten attended the Callanish weeklong retreat six weeks after her stem cell transplant for relapsed Hodgkin's lymphoma, a type of cancer most commonly diagnosed in young adults, and often curable. The transplant was Kirsten's only hope for a cure, since three different chemotherapy regimens had failed over the course of the previous year.

She had run a marathon soon after the month-long hospitalisation for the transplant and she said the twenty-six-mile run felt like a short walk in the park compared to the transplant. She had a lot to live for. She was only thirty-two and she and Ian, her husband of just two years, had promising careers and hopes for kids.

Kirsten's big blue eyes seemed locked open wide, reminding me of the shock in the eyes of a toddler whose doll has been snatched away by another child, the kind of shock that registers loss just before the wailing starts. Kirsten's skin was translucent, and her willowy body housed the fragility brought about by a month in the hospital and extra-high-dose chemotherapy – enough to kill her, had the stem cells not been infused back into her body as soon as her blood counts dropped to zero. Once they graft in the bone marrow the stem cells become the start of a new, hopefully cancer-free life.

Kirsten told me she always felt cold since the transplant. She spent most of the retreat week wrapped in a blanket over layers of clothes, tucked in on the couch by the fire.

The love and care, healthy food, massage, music, art-making, heartfelt conversations and walks in nature brought some life back to Kirsten. Over six days, she slowly began to emerge from her cocoon; her appetite improved, her skin brightened, and we began to get to know this peaceful warrior. She had grit and wit, and endless patience for listening to the stories of the other retreatants.

She called me four months after the retreat, her voice strong and animated.

'Janie, I have an idea. Can we meet to talk about it?'

I was pleased to hear from her.

'How about tomorrow afternoon for tea and a chat?' I asked.

'Sure, three o'clock?'

The next day, Kirsten hopped out of her navy Jeep with lightness in her step. Her blonde hair was long enough now to be swept up into a tiny ponytail high on her head, and her cheeks were rosy. She wore a summery blue-and-white blouse, a short down jacket and jeans. The only evidence of cancer was the one-inch scar to the right of her collarbone where her implanted intravenous device had been.

We sat on the couch in the group room with mugs of Earl Grey tea.

Kirsten launched in. 'Would you be interested in starting a writing series here at Callanish?' I knew Kirsten had been a journalist before cancer, and was excited to see her passion for what she did in life returning. 'Writing has been my lifeline throughout this nightmare with cancer,' she told me.

'Absolutely! I've thought about it many times, and just haven't put it into action. I must have been waiting for you,' I replied.

She told me her idea: 'We should have a maximum of fourteen people, once a week for eight weeks. Perhaps three hours a session, if you think people will have the energy. We could use the Amherst Writers' model of using prompts to help people focus on a topic. They can write for about thirty minutes, read if they want to, and then other group members can respond. They wouldn't critique the writing but rather speak of how the writing touched them, or challenged them.' She was bubbling with excitement.

'When shall we start?' I asked.

'Now?'

'Any ideas what to call the group?' I asked.

'Well, actually, I do!' She beamed. 'You already have Callanish Retreats and Callanish Reads, so what about Callanish Writes?'

'Looks like a new programme has just been born,' I said.

Cancer was nowhere to be seen as purpose radiated through Kirsten's glowing countenance.

We planned the first Callanish Writes series for spring 2008 and had a waiting list within a week of the announcement. Fourteen people registered, most with no previous writing experience. Well before the end of the first series, the writers asked for a second one.

The circle of fourteen Callanish writers gathered in the group room for the start of the second series in late fall of the same year. The fire crackled in the wood stove and rain pelted the skylights two storeys above our heads. Fleece blankets were wrapped around knees and journals lay closed on laps waiting to be opened to reveal the fresh writing. Kirsten shared a piece from her journal:

'After cancer set up camp in my body and I was on the road to supposed recovery, I was able to shed the itchy sweater of my "profes-sional self". I would never again have to ask the father of a drowned boy what his plans were now, or hold the microphone to the quiv-ering lips of a mother whose daughter had been murdered and ask her how she felt . . .'

Kirsten looked up at the group. 'My mom has been amazing, through all this. I couldn't have managed without her. She encouraged me to let go of my stressful career and said I'd find something else.' She reached for a tissue and dabbed her eyes, before finishing up: *'No — my future, however long it was going to be, was waiting to unfold in a new direction, and for me to walk toward it, one soft step at a time.'*

Kirsten closed her journal and let out a long breath. A few people shifted in their chairs as the reality of impermanence rustled through the group.

By late 2009, our third eight-week series of Callanish Writes was under way. A five-foot twisted tree branch lay on the coffee table, striking in its barrenness.

Kirsten loved choosing unique prompts that stimulated the writers to explore their lives in thought-provoking ways. She found poems and passages of prose that she thought would inspire creativity and also gathered up the writing at the close of each series and compiled anthologies that she got printed and bound for each group member to take home.

'Let's take about thirty minutes for writing today, and choose a time when you were at a crossroads, a branching point. Perhaps your life changed direction, by force of circumstance, or by choice. What was that like? How did you feel?' Kirsten said to the circle of fourteen. 'Use your five senses to describe that time in your life. May this tree branch be your muse.'

A quiet fell over the room as each writer faced the blank page.

'Just let the narrative write itself,' Kirsten said. 'It knows what it wants to say.'

Soon pens and pencils were heard moving across the page, scribing words that found their way from inside the mind of the writer out into the world for the first time. Minutes ticked by unnoticed.

After twenty-five minutes, Kirsten spoke. 'Take just another five minutes and find a place to pause. You may not be finished but that's okay.' Journals were closed one by one and the writers glanced around the room as though they were surfacing from a trance.

'Would anyone like to read to the group?' Kirsten asked. 'No pressure. Your work may be too fresh to be read aloud yet.' The group members looked down at what they had written, as if surprised by the marks on the page. 'Prudence may be sitting on your shoulder right now, judging you, but perhaps you can ignore her taunts and put-downs and read regardless.'

Kirsten had told the writers about Prudence, her nickname for the inner critic, and they had found the concept helpful for building confidence to write and to read aloud. The critic was a regular partici-pant in the minds of new writers in the early sessions of a series. Sometimes Prudence prevented the writer from reading, or provoked preambles such as: 'This isn't very good' or 'This is embarrassing to say out loud' or 'I'm just not as eloquent as the rest of you.'

As the weeks went by, Prudence was mostly forgotten about as each narrator found their own voice.

'I'll read,' said Marina.

Kirsten nodded for her to go ahead.

Marina read with ease and when she finished she looked down at her hands in her lap. Her cancer was not responding to chemotherapy and her children were still in elementary school.

Kirsten then asked the group, 'What stays with you about Marina's writing? What word or sentence stands out for you? What moved you? How did her writing touch your own experience of cancer?'

The group was asked not to evaluate the writing.

If one writer's work is considered 'wonderful, profound or well-written', it can evoke a sense of other writing being inferior. When responders articulate their own personal responses to the writing it often brings insight to the writer.

'I love the phrase "fire of living". It feels like that to me too, that the fire of life is both scary and exciting,' said Stephen, whose cancer had recently recurred. 'Having cancer is terrifying, the dry branch of your life could explode into flames with one small ember, and yet there is this *fire of living* too that has ignited a kind of urgency in my life. No time to waste. That's exciting – it wakes me up! Don't interpret this as meaning that cancer is a gift, though. I hate that overused phrase! It makes me want to re-gift the present to the sender.' He laughed.

'I'll read next,' said Yvonne, who'd been given a very poor prognosis nine months before. She surprised herself and her doctors by getting better, and she had no idea why. 'I've called my piece "Branching Off",' she said.

The palm reader says she knows how to read palms.
We look at my right hand.
My lifeline branches off very strongly
But also continues for a long while.
Was that branching-off cancer?

Or was it the decision to handle things in my life differently from my family of origin?
Do I believe I will live long?
Do I believe I am different?
Do I believe that what I did saved me?

Amara, a woman in her late sixties, hadn't yet spoken. In remission for two years from breast cancer, she considered herself cured. She pulled on the fingers of her left hand with her right hand, one finger at a time, and her joints popped as she spoke.

'Yvonne, it scares me to think we have that much control over the length of our lives. It means there might be something more I could or should be doing. I want to know your secret, but then it might not be mine,' Amara said.

'Your writing makes me hopeful, Yvonne,' said Kirsten. 'We never do know, do we, when we're going to die? I like the mystery of that because maybe my script is not yet written.'

Ten writers read, four chose not to. Vast spans of time and the tiniest moments were written about, and responded to, by a group of people grappling with the realities of living and dying.

The session ended with a poem for the road, read by Kirsten.

For the Record
by Kirsten Andersen

You arrived
tattered and torn
bursting at the seams
spilling forth
an account of this body.
Four long years
fourteen hundred and fifty-two days
narrated across thousands of pages
by countless doctors
in Vancouver
Montreal
Seattle
Texas
all describing the 'unfortunate young lady'
'an anxious thirty-two-year-old'
'with no history of illness'
'thin and pale'
'a sizeable mass in the chest'
'unusually aggressive disease'
'no known cure – worldwide'
'palliative chemo for this "tragic case".

Am I tragic?

These words have been dictated,
transcribed, typed and now delivered to me
in a ragged envelope,
arriving with the flyers and bills
lying beside me in bed this morning.
GPs, surgeons, oncologists, endocrinologists,
radiologists, hematologists,
all have had their way with my body,
its blood, its marrow, its developing cells,
telling a story
seemingly hopeless and futile
sad and tragic
until
now.

The fifth series had been planned for the fall 2010. Kirsten's cancer had returned. She was undergoing palliative treatment to try to stall progression of the disease, but it wouldn't be curative. Kirsten and I chose the theme of Time. The writing would focus on our relationships with the past, the future and the present moment. There were twelve returning writers and two new ones.

Kirsten and I worried whether she'd have enough energy to lead the group. Each morning for a week before the first session, Kirsten and I spoke on the phone. She was feeling terrible. The new chemotherapy

zapped every ounce of her energy, and she barely made
the journey from her bed to the couch every day.

Just a few hours before the first group, Kirsten
conceded defeat. The decision was a momentous one.
The writing group had become one of her main
reasons for getting up in the morning.

'I've been dreading that this cancer would eventually
stop me from doing what I love. I hate this disease.'

I could sense the wail beneath the fury.

'I hate it too, I really do. I'm so sorry you can't
come today.' I knew not to even try and make it better.
I listened while she continued.

'I'm scared I'll never be back to the group again.'
Her voice shook.

'I'm sure you are afraid. Fear does have a way of
shrinking the future. Let's get you through today
first,' I said.

'Yeah, okay. I'll take a nap now and then maybe
I'll try and write a bit – use the prompt we planned
for the group today.'

'By the way, you do know groups are mobile, right?
Remember when we took the reading group to Carol-
Anne's house when she couldn't get to Callanish?'

All the writers in the fifth series knew Kirsten and
feelings about her absence became our first writing
prompt that afternoon.

I wrote this poem for her:

For Kirsten, my friend and mentor

How can you be so present?
in this circle today,
in your absence?
Your body is missing,
but your heart and your spirit
are sitting right here beside me.
I can hear you and feel you
on the inside of me,
where you always live.

A couple of weeks after the fifth series ended, and just a month before Christmas, Kirsten agreed that a small group of writers she knew well could travel to her home for a one-off writing session. Everyone there knew she was dying. It turns out her mother hadn't known Kirsten was dying. After reading the story recently, she explained in an email:

'The truth is, though, that I didn't know. I never believed that she wasn't going to use her extraordinary tenacity to turn things around, to spring back into her life, even up to her very last day. I still (more than eight years later) have trouble truly acknowledging that she is gone and I can't use that word myself. I always refer to having "lost" her, because that is exactly what it feels like.'

The death of a child evokes its own narrative for every parent. I received an important teaching from this interaction with Kirsten's mother, one that has humbled me: I can never presume to know what any person faced with an unfathomable, unacceptable loss understands to be true.

It was a dark, gloomy afternoon when six of us were greeted by Finnegan, Kirsten and Ian's chocolate Lab, at the door of their cottage in Deep Cove. Kirsten sat on the couch in the living room. She had lost several pounds and her cheekbones were prominent under her blue-grey eyes. What little energy she had was being gifted to this gathering. She would likely pay for it for several days after.

'I can't tell you what it means to have you here. I have missed you all so much.' Her voice, though weak, carried the intensity of a woman who knew that time was precious. There were no dry eyes in the room as we registered being in the midst of an ending, one that shattered any hope for a future for Kirsten and her family.

'Well, let's write then,' she said. 'That's what you are here for! You know I can't tolerate too much weeping and wailing.' For her sake, we attempted a laugh.

We kept the writing time to ten minutes and then

we shared our writing as we always did. Each person read twice, and a few people responded.

Carol-Anne read her poem over the sound of her oxygen tank. Like Kirsten, she also knew that her time was limited.

At Kirsten's in Her White Room

We arrive after a bridge and slick rain-laden
    roads,
entry: white, calm, Mom, tea ready to go.
Cookies abound, all that matters is gathering
    now.
Kirsten is here, wrapped warm, semi-fragile,
yet ever so present.
It will be dark when we're done; it might be
    cold – wet.
Yet all that matters is we all arrived.
We are simple; it is simple, like your space, safe
    and white.
We know we are here, we have arrived – for you.
Kirsten, you are all that matters.

Each writer read, and each piece was a tribute to Kirsten, and a goodbye. On the way out, the writers stalled at the front door, stumbling to find the right words for the ending that was upon them. If we acknowledged that this was likely our last visit, would that convey to Kirsten that we were giving up hope? If we didn't acknowledge it as the last time we'd see each other, would we hurt Kirsten? Would saying 'Merry Christmas' be okay, knowing merry was likely not how this Christmas was going to be?

It's helpful at times like that to stay in the present and take the lead from the sick person.

'Thanks for coming all this way,' Kirsten said to the group, as they fumbled with boots and coats. 'Fingers crossed we'll meet here again. And if not, keep writing, okay? Merry Christmas, everyone,' Kirsten said, as brightly as she could muster. She had ensured a dignified goodbye.

Her shoulder blades protruded against the palms of my hands as I hugged her. 'You are very dear to me, and always will be,' I murmured into her ear. 'Thank you for everything.'

Three weeks later freezing rain thwacked my windshield as I drove across the Second Narrows Bridge, for what would turn out to be my last visit with Kirsten. I parked on the street, pushed open the car door against the weather and let myself in through the front door. Ian had told me not to knock, that he'd leave the door open for me.

The queen-sized bed filled the only bedroom of

their cottage, with its pocket view of the sea. All I could see of her was a wisp of blonde hair peeking out from under the mountainous white duvet.

I leaned towards the mound. 'Kirsten, Janie here. Ian said you might be up for a short visit,' I said.

Kirsten's face emerged from under the duvet. 'Nice,' she said, and flickered a smile.

'I can just sit here quietly while you rest, or read you some poetry?'

I pressed my hand gently on top of the duvet over where I thought her arm might be.

'Mmm, poetry please.'

'I brought you the fifth anthology,' I said.

I was so relieved that she would see the last book in the set of five she had envisioned three years before.

'Purple, I hoped it would be purple,' she whispered, as she looked at the book in my hand.

Kirsten had loved choosing the colours for the covers of each of the previous anthologies. She wanted the jacket colour to feel congruent with the words inscribed inside. I was glad she liked it.

I slid the chair closer to the bed and noticed the framed wedding photo in among the Kleenex, mouthcare sponges and lip balms on the bedside table.

I opened the slim, shiny purple book, *Callanish Writes: Volume V*, and flipped to page eleven. Kirsten had been too sick to lead any sessions in the fifth writing series but had insisted we write in her absence.

'We included a few poems we wrote for you in our new volume,' I said. 'I'd like to read MaryAnne's poem.'

MaryAnne, like Kirsten, was in her early thirties when she was diagnosed with cancer. She found writing to be therapeutic as she went through the rigours of treatment and attended as many of the writing sessions as she could.

Kirsten closed her eyes as I read.

> Lovely One
> by MaryAnne Brown
>
> Lovely one
> though you are far,
> yet you are near.
> Your never-ending poems
> whisper beautiful secrets
> to lead us forward.
> And we write
> to secure grace enough
> for us all,
> and for you.

Kirsten rolled over slowly to face me and opened her eyes, which still carried the presence of her spirit, though living in a body almost too weak to house it for much longer.

'Can I read you one last poem?' I asked. She nodded.

> To Kirsten
> by Laura Paul
>
> To you on the first day
> Of your fifth group
> Miss you
> Miss you lots today
> Our merry muse of words
> The twinkle, the shine
> As your love of words pours forth
> And flows to fill the space
> And takes us from laughter to tears
> And back again
> On the roundtrip
> Heartfelt journey of wonder and words
> With loving kindness to you.

My voice trembled. In the presence of Kirsten's life ending, love mixed with sorrow made it hard to speak. I closed the book and laid it on the top of her pile of books on her bedside table.

'Do you know Callanish Writes kept me going when

I doubted I could go on?' Kirsten said. 'It gave me the purpose I'd always been looking for and never could find.'

'I will miss you, my co-leader. You have taught me so much. It won't be the same without you.' My face was wet with sorrow. 'If I ever get a book written, I will dedicate it to you for believing in me as a writer.' I leaned forward to kiss her cool cheek goodbye.

Finnegan licked my hands as I pulled on my boots and let myself out of the front door. I noticed that Ian had fallen asleep on the couch in the living room.

Kirsten died at home under her mountainous white duvet on 7 February 2011.

Callanish Writes is thriving.

13

LOUISE: The Possibility of Forgiveness

Louise and I met for the first time in the summer-house set amongst an impressive stand of firs, a few minutes' walk uphill from the retreat centre. I thought Louise might prefer privacy for our initial conversation, rather than being among the other retreat participants, as I noticed she chose to sit alone at lunch.

Louise was diagnosed with a rare form of cancer at the age of thirty-five, and six months later it had spread to other organs. She'd been given a prognosis of less than a year then, but two years had passed by the time we found ourselves sitting together on a faded wooden bench under the canopy of the summerhouse. The sides of the octagonal structure were open to the forest and the cool air seeped in, low to the ground, as the late September day came to its close.

'What do you hope to get out of this week?' I asked.

Louise answered without lifting her eyes to meet mine. Her words were measured, as though they might give away incriminating evidence. I had seen the blanket of shame before, wrapping people up in a shroud of unworthiness.

'I didn't know where else to turn,' she said, her fingers tapping the side of the bench and her feet scuffing the worn floorboards. 'I've never really wanted to live, until now.' She paused for several seconds, as though she had to wait for the words to arise from deep inside the darkness. 'The cancer made me want to live; the irony of it all,' she said.

Louise had tried every healing modality she could find to cure her cancer: naturopathy, homeopathy, meditation, energy healing and faith healing, as well as conventional cancer treatments. No stone had been left unturned, except for the retreat. Louise hoped the week on retreat might unlock the key to her survival, regardless of my explanation during our initial phone conversation that the retreat is about healing, not curing. Often people need to focus their hope somewhere, and for Louise, it was on the retreat.

'I believe if I could deal with my past, then my body could heal. The memories take my life force, like vampires,' she said. Her shoulder-length brown hair, parted in the middle, hung straight and heavy, obscuring most of her face.

'Do you believe that your past caused your cancer?' I asked.

'Maybe,' she said. 'All through my adolescence and early twenties, I wanted to die. I left my family as soon as I could, at seventeen. Do you think a death wish can cause cancer?'

'Many people who have unbearable childhoods wish they could will themselves to die, to escape, but after thirty years in this work I have to say I believe cancer is mostly random, and the mind is not as powerful as we might like to think it is,' I said, feeling the flush of conviction warm my cheeks.

In fact, in the years since Louise died, some research studies have shown that there is an increased risk of illnesses, including cancer, in people who have experienced adversity in childhood, such as trauma, abuse and neglect. Louise's belief in her past having an impact on her cancer diagnosis was the motivation for healing. She knew what she was doing.

Louise looked up at me for the first time. A deep melancholy oozed from her flat grey eyes, but I noticed too that a flicker of connection moved across the space between us. In my experience, once the impetus to heal from an abusive childhood is triggered it can move people out of the inertia of self-blame and into the possibility of freedom.

That evening Louise told the group about her life since her cancer diagnosis. She spoke of the ten-hour surgery and its painful aftermath and described in detail how sick she was during the year of chemotherapy, and how she went to every appointment at the cancer centre alone.

Each time Louise told another instalment of her story, group members nodded with concern and encouragement for her to keep going. They knew not to interrupt her with advice, questions or platitudes.

After about half an hour Louise said, 'I didn't think anyone would ever stay long enough to hear the whole horrible story.'

Over the next five years Louise became a regular client in my counselling office, and a participant in many of the support groups at our centre. About two years after we met, towards the end of the session, Louise told me she was an incest survivor.

'He put poison in my body and caused my cancer and though I've tried to get rid of it, it's still there,' she said. 'I guess what I'm saying is that having cancer now is my fault, for not trying harder to be free of it.' She then stood up slowly. 'I've got to go now.'

The starkness of her conviction took my breath away.

'Thank you for telling me, Louise,' I said as she opened the door. 'Call me if you need to before we see each other next week, okay?' She nodded and closed the door softly behind her.

Louise worked hard to heal her broken spirit, even as her body gradually succumbed to cancer. She grieved the parents and the childhood she never had, and raged against her loss of innocence. She learned to forgive herself for all the ways she had mistreated her body and she released her guilt that the abuse had somehow been her fault. Gradually, Louise began to describe an inner aliveness she felt inside her ailing body. She said her spirit must have reawakened after a long sleep.

At forty-three, eight years after she was expected to die, Louise was nearing the end of her life. She had been admitted to the palliative care unit several times for pain management and had started to give away her possessions to her closest friends.

Early one morning I received an urgent voice message from Louise. 'I woke up last night and heard a voice in my head: *You have to confront your father before you die.* You gotta be kidding me, I thought. I can't do that. Way too scary and he'd probably kill me,' she said. Her voice was shaking. 'But Janie, I know now I can't die with this terrible secret in my heart and in my family. I have to tell the truth. Will you help me?' she asked.

'Of course I'll help you,' was my automatic response. A torrent of feelings and questions rushed through me on the back of my commitment to help Louise confront her father. *What if he denies the abuse? What if he refuses to talk? What if he accepts responsibility?* I felt afraid and hopeful at the same time. I also knew I would need help from another therapist with more experience in interventions around sexual abuse than I had.

I called Susan, a psychologist I knew well, who had worked for years with incest survivors, and the three of us spent hours together over the next several weeks planning and practising how we would safely do what had become imperative: Louise would speak her truth to her father.

Louise had maintained a distant relationship with her parents in Alberta, visiting with them once or twice a year, but never staying in their home. The abuse had never been discussed in the family. She emailed to invite them to a meeting in Vancouver to discuss end-of-life issues. They agreed to come.

* * *

Louise and I entered the therapy room. Susan had arrived early to settle Louise's parents before we arrived. Louise nodded briefly at her parents, who sat across the room from each other. Louise chose the chair closest to the door, and furthest from her father.

While Susan set the stage for the meeting, with ground rules about listening and not interrupting, I made my assessment, one quick glance at a time. Louise's father was about six feet tall and skinny, wearing jeans, a plaid shirt and a baseball cap loose over his short-cropped grey hair. His body leaned forward, his gaze to the floor, concentrated. Louise's mother, a short stout woman in her sixties, was dressed in a faded blue cardigan over brown corduroys and stared listlessly at her hands clasped together in her lap. I wondered if she was listening, or whether she had taken herself off to a made-up place, as people who are hurting do.

Louise had written letters she intended to read, first to her father, then to her mother. She had rehearsed the reading several times, a few days before, and had tried to anticipate every possible reaction. We had arranged for another colleague to sit in the waiting room in case her father flew into a rage, as he'd so often done when Louise was a child.

Louise looked at me as if to say, *Here I go*. I smiled

encouragement at her. She then spoke the words she had waited most of her life to say. Her voice was clear and strong.

'*Dad, what I'm going to say to you today is for me, not for you. I need to let go of a family secret before I die, and I need to tell you that what you did to me cost me my life.*' Louise paused for a few breaths, looking down at her paper. '*You abused me physically and sexually and I've hated you and wished you dead for what you did to me. I'm the one who got cancer and I'm going to die. It doesn't seem fair. You should be the one to get cancer.*'

Louise looked up at him briefly then, likely checking that she was still safe. He continued to look at the floor. Her mother rocked slightly from side to side, her eyes flicking from right to left in sync with her body movements.

The room felt like it had been waiting a long time to hold this moment of potential healing, and I hoped its four walls could hold enough safety. I held my breath and focused on Louise, trying to push my support through the air towards her, willing her to continue, praying there would be no explosion from her father.

Louise continued, gaining confidence with each sentence. '*I lived in fear every day of my life because of you. I wanted to die, to get away from you. I had no self-confidence and no friends. You judged everything I said and did, and you never once said you were proud of me. The life I've built up around me now,*

*with my circle of friends, has nothing to do with you. I did it myself.
I like myself now, but it has taken me years of therapy, and a commitment to myself I never knew I had.'*

There was more of Louise in the room now,
expanding to fill its corners. She sat taller in the chair
with every word spoken. Louise's father had not
looked up. His body was frozen in place, the stillness
concealing his reaction. Her mother had stopped
rocking, which I hoped meant she was less afraid. I
wondered if she might even feel relieved that the truth
was now out in the open.

The next letter was for her mother.

Louise spoke in between sobs. *'Mom, how could you?
How could you let him do this to me? You are as much to blame as
him.'* Louise threw a look of disdain at her father. *'You
must have known what he was doing. And if you didn't, then what
is wrong with you?'* Her crying had stopped and her voice
grew louder. *'You should be ashamed of yourself. You've never
been a mother to me; you've never cuddled me or kissed me, or told
me you loved me. I feel sorry for you. I know you told me you were
abused as a child but that's not good enough. All the more reason
for you to protect your children.'*

Louise was shaking now. I leaned towards her and
placed my right hand firmly on her forearm. Louise's
mother now looked like she was well ensconced in
her faraway land. She had a faint smile on her face,
and her gaze shifted from her lap to the window and

back again in quick succession, over and over again. She likely wouldn't remember any of this. Dissociation is a coping strategy for when reality inflicts too much pain on the psyche.

Louise put the letters down. 'That's it,' she said, looking at me. The colour had seeped out of her already-pale face and she looked exhausted. Before the meeting, Louise told me that she wanted to read the letters and then go home. She didn't want to get pulled into conversation.

What happened next surprised us. Louise's father lifted his head and looked at her. 'Can I respond?' he asked in a soft, broken voice. Louise nodded her assent and looked at her lap. Her hands were clenched tightly. I deepened the pressure of my hand on her arm to convey my reassurance she could receive his words, or stop him if necessary.

'I've waited many years to say this to you, Louise. I wanted to but I couldn't. Maybe I didn't want to accept what I'd done.'

He paused for a moment as though waiting for courage to press him forward. I heard Louise take in a deep breath. She was hopeful.

'What happened should never have happened and I'm sorry for what I did, sorrier than you will ever know. I will never forgive myself for this, and I cannot expect to be forgiven.'

Louise lifted her eyes and locked in with her father's.

'Dad, I will never love you, nor forgive your actions, but in time I may be able to forgive you,' she said. 'Not yet, but for the first time in my life it feels possible.'

Louise's burden had been laid down at the feet of a man and a woman who had inherited ways of parenting that violated contracts of trust. She hoped that her courage might help stop the legacy of violence and worthlessness that had been passed down through generations. Louise had completed what she intended to: the secret was no longer hidden inside the family, or inside her. Turning towards me, Louise nodded for us to leave.

A few months after Louise confronted her father, her cancer began to recede. She put on weight and became interested in life again. Her scans showed that her cancer had not progressed. In fact, it was shrinking. She graduated from the palliative care programme, not something that happens often. When I asked her why she thought the cancer had receded, she answered, 'I don't really know, but maybe it's because I released the poison.'

Louise lived for five more years after the meeting with her family. Those years were filled with good life. She hiked the North Shore Mountains, which she never thought she would traverse again, and asked her friends to return some of the possessions she'd given them, thinking she was going to die.

IV.

SURRENDERING TO THE SPACIOUS HEART

*'The heart that
breaks open can
contain the
whole universe.'*
—JOANNA MACY

M any people feel supported by the teachings of spiritual traditions in their dying, and others who do not adhere to a specific spiritual belief system sometimes find ways to put their lived experience into a larger perspective. An expanded perspective often appears at unexpected moments, or in dreams, and the effect of putting one's own individual story into the collective can be both uplifting and calming.

I remember many moments of expanded awareness in my life, and they comfort me. I had a dream two nights before my father died that I was walking very slowly arm-in-arm with him up a winding forest path through a series of switchbacks. The feeling was that I was taking him somewhere, to a place where I knew we would be parting. Once we neared the top of the mountain, I could hear singing and I knew we were nearly there. As we entered a clearing, I saw a long-time mentor of mine, Dolores Krieger, coming towards us smiling.

'Ahh,' she said, 'you are here!'

She looked at Dad, nodding, and then to me and said, 'Thank you.'

I gave Dad a hug and then my mentor took him by the arm and turned. I knew I had delivered my father to where he needed to go next, and my work was done. This dream made sense to me after I awoke: the work of caring for him in his dying was almost done. Somehow dreaming that he would be safe and loved by a mentor of mine when we parted released me to let him go. I felt deeply at peace during those last two days of his life.

Awe and wonder at the beauty and power of nature, or the tender moments between two people who know that life is truly transitory, or a ceremony of beauty to honour those we love, can remind us that we are connected to a world which participates in the cycles of creation and destruction, beginnings and endings, and can help us to realise just how excruciatingly beautiful our existence on this earth is.

Many people with cancer have told me stories about how nature interacted with them at times when they were struggling. A hummingbird, a raven or a pod of orcas inspired them when they were frightened; a giant spider's web shimmering in the early morning dew calmed anxiety, or sunbeams bursting through fresh green leaves to the forest floor comforted their sorrows.

Unexpected encounters in nature have stopped me in my tracks too, and have shaken me out of an entrenched state of mind or heart. My mood has been altered by moments when a creature, a bird, a changing sky or a white-capped ocean drew me out of inner turmoil into the world with its ever-changing vistas and perspectives.

Once, as I was walking alone through a forest, mourning the death of a close friend, I looked up to see a great-horned owl high in an ancient ponderosa pine. Looking down at me, he gave me a slow wink, as if to say, *We're all in this together*. Of course, I understood he was only blinking, but his comradely wink gave me such delight that for a few moments I forgot my broken heart.

An enormous tortoise walked towards me in the dry wash of the Californian desert one afternoon while I was on a ten-day silent meditation retreat. After listening to a prayer for the healing of the earth, I left the meditation hall weeping inconsolably for the horrors we humans have inflicted on our planet. As I walked across land scorched by the sun, between sobs, I mumbled, 'I'm sorry, earth, I'm so sorry.'

Out of nowhere an ancient tortoise trundled up

to me, stopped about two feet from where I stood and looked me directly in the eye. After a few moments of holding my gaze, the tortoise turned and slowly walked away.

Many cultures see the turtle as a symbol of Mother Earth and I imagined the desert tortoise was saying to me, *The earth is okay. Don't worry so much*. I was deeply comforted by the surprise of those unexpected moments that allowed my deep sorrow for the planet to be held in a larger perspective.

The seven stories in this final section, *Surrendering to the Spacious Heart*, describe how connecting to a larger view can allow for a deep understanding of our inter-connectedness with all people, close and far, living and dead, who have also had to, or will have to, encounter dying. We all belong to that global commu-nity and can draw strength and comfort from it if we open our hearts wide enough to recognise its enor-mous presence.

14

PHILIP: The Rightness of Everything

Philip and I cycled abreast into the large grey raincloud that enveloped the forest road. Conifers towered above us and salal on the verges shone bright green in the rain. The other riders in our training group for the 2013 Whistler Gran Fondo were ahead, out of sight. Philip had slowed down to wait for me.

'It's safer to lean away from the corners when it's wet, Janie,' he said.

I wasn't used to the thin, no-tread tyres on my new road bike yet.

'You're doing great for a beginner roadie.'

I glanced sideways at him, daring to take my eyes off the road for a moment.

'You're not doing so bad yourself for someone on chemotherapy,' I replied.

Philip and I met when he attended a young adult support group, just after he finished his first round of cancer treatment. He spoke in his soft, speedy Irish brogue about the devastation of having his life shattered by cancer.

'It strips you of everything you believe in, everything you think you can count on.'

Nods of assent had rippled around the circle. Eighteen young adults in their twenties and thirties were candid about having been diagnosed with cancer and being catapulted out of lives that were just getting going. Philip and Rima were the only two in the circle that night with Stage IV cancer that was considered incurable. Rima lived with breast cancer that had spread to her liver and bones, and was enrolled in a palliative care programme. They gravitated towards each other at the end of the evening.

A month before the birth of his first child, Philip had learned that the original cancer in his nasal passages, after three years in remission, had spread to his lungs. The oncologist told him he would only have a few months to live. In my experience, younger people with cancer often live longer than their doctors predict, perhaps because the doctors base their prognoses on older people with cancer, for whom they have greater numbers and hence more accurate statistics.

On this damp Sunday morning in April, Philip was two months into chemotherapy and back on his bike for the first time since his re-diagnosis.

Philip had been raised in Hong Kong by his mother Wong Yuen Wai, who had worked in a plastic flower factory since she was eleven years old, his father Lee Siu Ming, a postman, and his grandmother, who cared for him for many hours a day while his parents worked. The family of six crowded into a two-bedroom high-rise apartment, and when Hong Kong was to be returned to China in the 1990s they decided to emigrate to Dublin. Philip was twelve years old.

He started cycle racing in 1999, at the age of fourteen, and travelled around Ireland with his coach, becoming a top junior cyclist. By nineteen, his competitive cycling was over. His coach told him he wasn't good enough to make it to the top. Philip only raced again eight years later, when he cycled in L'Étape du Tour, the world's largest amateur cycle race, in the French Alps in 2012. By then, he had emigrated to Canada with his Irish wife Emma, and had recovered from his first cancer diagnosis.

I hesitated when he'd proposed forming a team to ride in the Whistler Gran Fondo on 7 September 2013 as a fundraiser for Callanish. For eighteen years our charity had avoided holding community events that exclude people who are not physically strong enough to participate. I carried out a mini-survey of several members who were living with advanced cancer and asked them how they felt about a Callanish cycling team riding to raise money in a sporting event which, by its nature, excluded most ill people.

The responses were unanimously positive:

'If you're lucky enough to have your physical health, use it for good.'

'Celebrate your health. I wish I had when I was healthy, when I took my health for granted.'

'Ride for all of us. We'll get pulled along in your draught.'

We received full endorsement for Team Callanish.

A volunteer organising committee was struck up to help the team reach its fundraising goal and to support riders in their 122-kilometre cycle from Vancouver to Whistler along the Sea to Sky Highway, with an elevation gain of 1,900 metres.

My response was immediate when Philip suggested I ride myself.

'Are you kidding me? I'm too old. I don't have a road bike. I'm not competitive, and those hills are unthinkable.' The excuses rolled off my tongue.

Later that night I thought more about Philip's proposition.

What takes me out of my comfort zone? When do I tackle the impossible? Could I do it?

For close to thirty years I'd listened to people with cancer tell me about their challenges, and watched them set goals for themselves, ones that seemed unattainable. I'd seen people step towards their fear with courage, not permitting it to rob them of their will.

My first thought when I woke the next morning was: *I have to try. If Philip and Rima are riding while on chemotherapy for advanced cancer, then I must ride. The worst that could happen is that I wouldn't finish or I'd get injured; one would hurt my pride, the other my body.*

I picked up the phone. 'Okay, Philip. I am going to try to ride to Whistler with the team. You and Rima have inspired me to do my best, but I *am* terrified.'

'Hooray for you! No need to be scared. All you have to do is train consistently for the next five months and you'll finish,' Philip said.

All I have to do. I repeated this phrase many times during the following months of training.

I emailed our community to ask for interested riders, hoping for thirty but with no idea if there'd be any takers. Within a few weeks we had our team of thirty: those who had survived cancer or were living with it; family members of people who had survived or died of cancer; staff members and supporters of Callanish. Most of us were rookie roadies.

* * *

Twice a week from March to September, rain or shine, Team Callanish ventured out onto the British Columbia roads to build up power and endurance, often accompanied by Coach Philip.

'Janie, try to keep your cadence up,' Philip said as we climbed the ramp to the peak of the Lions Gate Bridge.

'What's cadence?'

'Cadence is the revolution of your pedals. Lower your gear to increase your revolutions per minute.'

It was a slow and steep learning curve.

During the spring months, Philip's cancer responded well to chemotherapy. The lung tumours shrank but so did his stamina. He tired easily on training rides, and often turned back early.

'You're all doing so well. Can't believe the improvement. Hope to see you next week!' he called out over his shoulder as his body and bicycle turned around on the road, as one. Beneath his helmet his hair was thinning.

My strength and confidence grew over the weeks of training. I started to enjoy my bike. Instead of thinking that it controlled me, that without warning it might divert me into oncoming traffic, or over an embankment into the ocean, I began to take charge. On the homecoming stretch from West Vancouver through Stanley Park, I reached sixty kilometres per hour.

I had never been one to linger in stores, but I developed strange new shopping behaviours. I stood in front of shelves of electrolyte tablets, deciding which flavour would be most palatable in my water bottle. I pondered interminably which energy bar to buy: the mint chocolate, the fig date or the oatmeal raisin. I tottered up the aisles of Mountain Equipment Co-op in my cleats, looking at skin-tight cycling shorts and jerseys, wondering which ones might cover up midlife bulges.

The day before the big ride my phone rang.

'Hi Janie, Philip here. Are you ready?' he asked in a subdued tone.

'Not much I can do now, Philip, is there?' I said. 'I may as well try to enjoy myself. What's up?'

'Well, I just left the cancer clinic, and the news is not good.'

My chest tightened. 'Tell me.'

'The cancer is growing again. The oncologist said I'll have to go on a different chemo, or I won't live to see Finn grow up,' Philip said. 'She was pretty brutal.'

The fact that the cancer was growing while Philip was on chemotherapy meant it was aggressive.

I took a big breath to settle my racing mind. Oncologists sometimes don't know where to locate hope in apparently hopeless situations.

'I don't know whether to come this weekend. I'm so frightened, and I don't want to bring the team down,' Philip said, his voice shaking. 'Does this mean I'm a goner?'

The team would be devastated. I bought some time and let the news fall deeper inside me. 'Philip, what did your oncologist say about whether you should ride or not?'

'She said it won't make any difference.'

I opened my mouth, not sure what was going to emerge. I wanted to scream at the cruelty of life, rage against the barbaric disease as I sometimes do in private. But I have learned to trust the relationship I've built with a person over months or years, and hope that helpful words will find their way to the surface.

'You could have received this news on Monday, two days from now, instead of today. If so, you would have come and had a wonderful weekend with everyone, oblivious of the growing cancer,' I said. 'Enjoy your weekend away with your family. You'll feel awful if you stay home. Come and be with people who love you, and who rely on you. Even if cancer's got hold of parts of your body, don't let it take your spirit.'

Philip sighed. I hoped I had reassured him that he was welcome to come, however he was feeling.

'Okay, Janie. I'll talk to Emma and let you know what we decide.' He hung up.

Philip left a voicemail later that evening.

'We're in the car. Good luck. See you at the finish line.'

At six a.m. that September Saturday, twenty-eight members of Team Callanish joined over four thousand other riders in the morning half-light on West Georgia Street. A light rain was falling. It was easy to spot each other in the crowd, with our sky-blue team jerseys bearing the names of people we had chosen to honour on the ride embossed onto one sleeve. The air was electric. Five months of training would pay off, or not.

Philip and Rima were riding the Medio Fondo, which started in Squamish, and although it was half the distance of the Gran Fondo, it was more than double the elevation gain of the Vancouver–Squamish section. The long, steep hill climbs would demand a lot of their compromised lungs.

Philip's voice echoed in my mind:

Eat breakfast an hour before you leave the house. Complex carbo-hydrates last longer in your system. Pack energy bars and wine gums in your jersey pockets for quick sugar boosts, and two full water bottles, one with electrolytes and the other with plain water. You'll need to fill them at most of the rest stops to keep well hydrated.

West Georgia Street moved like a conveyor belt. Riders were slow at first and then picked up speed; hundreds of riders rounded the bend onto the Stanley Park Causeway. The flashing lights of an ambulance ahead were foreboding. Information rippled through the group.

'The road is slippery,' people warned. 'Someone's gone down.'

Team Callanish crossed Lions Gate Bridge just as dawn broke along the eastern horizon. The ocean was far below us and the North Shore Mountains revealed themselves slowly under rising rainclouds.

We geared up and turned right, en masse, pushing up Taylor Way, the enormous hill that had scared me from day one. To my surprise, the road was lined on both sides with people. Children shook cowbells and noisemakers, and old people bundled up in down coats under umbrellas called out, 'You can do it! Way to go!'

I believed them and waved my thanks.

I geared up, rounded the curve high above the village of Horseshoe Bay and took in my first glimpse of Howe Sound. I thought of all the hundreds of people who donated to support our team, and the volunteers who were already up at the Brew Creek Centre near Whistler, preparing a feast for after the ride. I thought of family and friends waiting at the finish line to welcome us. I remembered the people for whom we were riding: those with cancer who had died, those who had survived, and all their family members who had endured their own burdens from cancer. I glanced down at the name *Bill Brown* on my sleeve. My sisters and brother and I had bought our father a red mountain bike for his sixtieth birthday, and I imagined he would have been proud of me. I thought of Rima and Philip ahead of me on the road and wished them well. My heart brimmed with something unexpected. Instead of fear and doubt, I felt love and gratitude.

We cruised past the first rest stop, well fuelled, and pulled into the second at Britannia Beach, the fifty-one-kilometre mark. The rain had stopped and the ocean reflected the metallic grey of giant cumulus clouds. The town of Squamish was bright and cheerful, with crowds of waving locals lining the highway. Several kids jumped up and down under a home-painted sign that read *CRISPY BACON HERE!* Bare hands held out rashers of bacon to any cyclist close enough to grab one.

The hill up to the Alice Lake rest stop was daunting, eight kilometres of 8 per cent gradient. Just as I was flagging, a mariachi band on the right-hand side of the road caught my eye. Three men in full Mexican costume stood side-by-side on the grassy verge, two strumming guitars and one playing a violin. Strains of 'La Cucaracha' serenaded us up the rest of the hill to rest stop number three, at seventy-three kilometres.

Two more rest stops for fresh orange segments and water bottle refills, and then on to Powerline Hill, the last major climb before Whistler.

At Whistler Creekside we pulled off to wait for the rest of our group of eight to cycle the last five kilometres together into Whistler Village. Our timing chips, firmly attached to our front forks, didn't matter any more. We would make it in just over seven hours and that was good enough. Two of our group had slowed to a snail's pace, likely due to hypoglycaemia, and two others had major leg cramps. All of us were tired and hungry, but spirits were soaring.

Turning the final corner, we glimpsed the colourful cycling advertisements flanking the exit ramp and the Gran Fondo banner flapping high over the finish line. As we cruised down the last hill, a line of sky-blue jerseys came into view on the left side of the road, and then we heard the full force of the Callanish roar. Many from the team, including Rima and Philip, whooped and hollered as our group of nine flew across the finish line.

Coach Philip beamed as he hugged me.

'You did it, Janie! Well done!'

'How did you do?' I asked.

'I can't believe it, but I placed seventh in the Men's Medio. It was an incredible ride. I will tell you the whole story later, over a beer.'

Several weeks later at a farewell tea for Philip, who was returning to live in Dublin, to be closer to family, he told the story of his Medio ride.

An elder from the Squamish Nation had opened the ride with a song for courage and safety. In a group of two hundred riders, Rima and Philip set off together in honour of their survivorship and friendship. At the two-kilometre mark Rima said, 'Now off you go, Philip, you've got to get ahead of your fucking cancer.'

Rima said that seeing Philip accelerate up the hill was like watching a heron take off from the shore.

'It was so beautiful to see him at one with his bike.'

Something extraordinary happened to Philip that day on the road. Even with the terrible news he had received the day before, instead of riding with bitterness and anger, he felt only love.

'I rode to conquer the hurts of cancer, not just in my body but in my heart,' he said. 'I had to accept that even though cancer has taken me away from the life I loved, it has given me a different life, one I've got to come to terms with.'

He was filled with awe at the beauty of the west

coast and felt deeply connected to the rest of the team members on the road.

'It sounds weird perhaps, but a raven looked me directly in the eye and it pierced me with the rightness of everything. It reassured me that everything was going to be okay, no matter what happens. I felt at peace for the first time in my life,' he said. 'And I continue to feel that way today. I feel reconnected to my spirit.'

A few months after the ride, Philip, his wife Emma and their son Finn moved back to Dublin for what would end up being the last year of his life. He spent several months cycling the Irish roads, until the cancer finally took the energy he needed for riding.

We kept in touch via Skype every few weeks until our final conversation when he was living in the hospice near his home. He told me that day that after many months of remembering his new-found connection to his spirit, he had slipped into darkness. He felt anxious and afraid about dying, and worried about how Emma and Finn and his parents would cope without him. Although he practised his beloved Qigong in the hospice garden every day when he had the strength, he had lost his larger perspective about life.

Although more than a year had gone by, I suggested we recall together the details of the day the team cycled to Whistler. We reminisced and shared our stories of the months of training and then the phone call that came on the day of the ride, relaying to Philip that his cancer was back. I asked him to remember the feeling of deciding to come to Whistler rather than choosing to stay home, the moment when he didn't let cancer take a front seat.

As he recalled the details of his decision, and the story of his personal ride and encountering the raven, I noticed Philip's voice had lifted and the expression on his face was brighter. Through the storytelling he reconnected himself to the team, to his will, and to his spirit.

Philip died peacefully a few days after that conversation and Team Callanish honoured him by riding together with a photograph of Coach Philip attached to our handlebars. His voice still coaches us as we tackle those steep hills, preparing for our next big fundraising ride.

15

RONALD AND MARCO:
Growing the Heart

R onald and Marco met in their early twenties in
Ontario, and when Marco's family shunned him
for being gay they moved to British Columbia, where
they married, chose a shared surname and bought their
first home. When I met them, they had been together
for thirty-eight years.

Marco stepped out of the driver's seat onto the
gravel parking lot of the retreat centre, his dark curly
hair framing his rugged Italian face.

'We made it! I'm the chauffeur dropping him off!'
He grabbed me for a brief hug before walking around
the Cadillac to open the passenger door. Marco's
warmth permeated the air between us, and although
we had not met before that moment, I felt like I'd
known him my whole life.

'We are here, my darling,' he said to Ronald.

A pale long-fingered hand extended out of the car and grasped Marco's sleeve. Ronald's perfectly oval hairless head emerged slowly and once his legs reassured him they'd hold him up, he raised his head and looked at me. An enormous grin opened up moments before large teardrops ran through the grey stubble on his chin.

'I can't believe I'm here,' he said, as he leaned his withered frame towards me for a hug.

The following morning, during the first group session, we focused on the theme of the weeklong retreat: Finding Meaning at the End of Life. I shared a teaching I had received during a meditation retreat from Zoketsu Norman Fischer, a Soto Zen priest. He talked about the fact that when we reach the end of our lives, and our bodies are no longer functioning well, we will likely still have access to the qualities that emanate from our hearts. He wasn't describing the condition of our physical hearts at the end of life, rather the feelings we often associate with heartfelt expression. The Buddhist teachings of the Brahmaviharas describe various contemplative practices to deepen qualities of the heart, such as kindness, compassion, appreciative joy and equanimity.

Ronald gasped when he heard this teaching. 'That's

it. My purpose at this stage of my life is to grow my heart. Marco will like that!'

He leaned forward in his armchair, eyes bright with curiosity.

'There are four primary qualities of the heart, according to the Buddhist teachings,' I said. 'No matter how ill the body is, we can choose to be more loving and kind towards ourselves, and towards other people. This first brahmavihara, translated from the Sanskrit *Mettā*, means "loving kindness".'

Ronald nodded enthusiastically.

'Second, we can develop our compassion, or *Karunā*, which is described as the natural arising of empathy in response to another person's suffering. The third primary quality of the heart is joy, or *Mudita,* which can arise surprisingly and spontaneously, sometimes in the midst of great suffering. Finally, we can develop more equanimity, or *Upekkhā*, an accept- ance of how things are, whether we like or dislike the circumstances of our lives,' I said.

The brahmavihara meditation practices Ronald learned during the retreat helped him to make a vital decision about chemotherapy. It had been causing increasing weakness and fatigue over the previous three months, and in spite of the treatment, the cancer was progressing. Directing loving-kindness towards himself during the *Mettā* practice made him realise that to continue to put chemotherapy into his failing body was unkind. He recognised that his fear was the driving force behind continuing treatment.

In the last evening group, Ronald spoke about his decision. 'I know that when I stop treatment, I will need to face my death head-on. I can't hide behind the minuscule chance that the chemo will put me into remission again,' he said. 'Stopping chemo feels like being kind to my poor body. And Marco will be relieved, not having to drive me back and forth to the cancer clinic, so it's kinder to him too.'

Ronald proclaimed that each day would now be for loving and living, no matter how many days he had left.

'Marco and I have been together for thirty-eight years. He will have to live off that love when I'm gone, so I'm going to generate as much love between us, and around us, from now until the day I take my last breath.'

Travelling into Vancouver to visit our centre for counselling and to attend support groups became increasingly difficult for Ronald in the months following the retreat, so Maryliz and I planned to visit Ronald and Marco in their home, about a forty-minute drive away.

Home visits are an integral component of our

programme so that people who are too ill to travel to see us can maintain support from our team, if they wish to. A closeness inevitably develops between us and our clients over the months and sometimes years. We must continually practise staying open and loving while anticipating the loss of people who become very dear to us.

We arrived at Ronald and Marco's home around one o'clock on a chilly Sunday in May. They were standing on the front doorstep when we pulled up outside their bungalow, which was set into the curve of a cul-de-sac. A faded folk-art sign hung on the wall to the right of the glass-inlaid front door. '*Bienvenuto*,' it read. 'Welcome.'

Ronald's grey knitted cardigan was at least two sizes too big and his pants were drawn in tight with a belt. Marco held him up as though Ronald belonged tucked in against his wide strong chest, with his arm firm around his husband's diminishing frame. Smile lines fanned out around the eyes of both men, whittled by lives of kindness. They welcomed us with hugs.

As we passed through the living room to the kitchen, I noticed that the dining-room table was set with Wedgwood, fine silver cutlery, crystal wine goblets and white linen napkins. Yellow tulips bowed low from a tarnished silver vase in the centre of the table. I assumed that Marco and Ronald were organised in advance for a dinner party they would be having later that evening and was glad Ronald thought he'd have the stamina to entertain.

Marco handed us both a small glass of sherry. 'You can't say no, okay?' he laughed. '*Salute. Cin-cin.*' We raised our glasses and clinked.

After a slow walking tour of the nooks and crannies of their home, filled with large colourful oil paintings, travel mementos and photographs that spanned their life together, Ronald asked, 'We assume you will accept our invitation for Sunday lunch?'

Any attachment to a schedule for the rest of the day dissolved as Maryliz and I glanced at each other and nodded. Marco squeezed my arm.

'It's our turn to spoil you now.'

He headed into the kitchen, with its bright white cupboards and equally bright white linoleum floor, and called, 'Talk amongst yourselves. Ronald, you've got loads of stories to tell them.'

As Marco bustled around the kitchen, Ronald told us about their life together. 'It wasn't easy to come out as gay men in those days, not like it is now, but we just couldn't live in the closet, and except for Marco's family most of our old friends weren't surprised when we told them we were in love,' he said. 'They were happy for us.' Conversation drifted back and forth between us with ease.

'Lunch is served,' Marco cried from the dining room.

What I assumed was the main course turned out to be the appetiser – traditional meat lasagne stacked high on the plate. Ronald poured Valpolicella into the crystal and raised his glass. 'Here's to love,' he toasted.

A steaming platter of braised steak, caramelised onions and mashed potatoes was served next, followed by a crisp romaine salad with cherry tomatoes and slices of avocado on top. The chocolate cheesecake smothered in whipped cream for dessert was accompanied by espresso coffee and flaming Sambuca.

'I feel like royalty,' I said.

'It's our turn to give back!' Marco yelled from the kitchen. He refused to let us help serve or take our dishes through. When he sat down to eat with us, he told us his stories about his love of Italian art, and music, and of course Ronald.

Marco wept when he spoke of his family's rejection of his homosexuality. He wiped his eyes frequently on his now-crumpled napkin. Ronald reached for his hand across the table, through the drooping yellow tulips.

Marco continued. 'Being from a first-generation Italian Catholic family was tough. Two men living together is a sin, even though I told them: "It's not a choice. I was born this way. Please understand that it's exactly the same love as you feel for each other." They refused to speak to me after that, told me I was no longer their son.' He clenched Ronald's hand tighter. 'That's why our chosen family, like you two and your team, means the world to us both.'

We could have been sitting in dappled sunshine at a white-tablecloth-clad tavola under olive trees in Tuscany, with a bottle of local vino partially drunk and a bowl of pasta with fresh parmigiana steaming in front of us, having a timeless conversation about love and loss, friendship and family.

Around four o'clock, Ronald told us that he had to rest. A double bed had been set up in the den off the dining room. The stairs to the master bedroom had become insurmountable.

'Come on in,' Ronald called out from the den. 'I'm not shy.'

When we entered the small den, Marco was gently tugging the grey cardigan off Ronald's bony shoulders. The pale blue Adidas t-shirt underneath had been ironed carefully. The bed took up almost the entire room, with just enough space to squeeze around either side. An antique dresser sat under the window, topped with a multitude of framed photographs, and all four walls were covered in Marco's art.

Marco looked over at us. 'I can't bear to be in our

big bed upstairs without him, so I sleep here too,' he said, as he pulled the white cotton duvet up over Ronald's shoulders. 'I'll be so lonely when he's gone.' The loneliness seemed to enter the room then, vast and inescapable, an unwelcome companion for the rest of Marco's life.

Not everyone is able to bring the future into the present like Marco did, out loud, acknowledging the loss that was to come for him. The openness between these two men showed me how willing and comfortable they must have been to feel the accompanying emotions that inevitably follow such a pronouncement, for both of them.

Maryliz leaned forward. 'Ronald, shall I play some music while you rest? I brought the ocarina, your favourite. Janie may even give you a foot massage, if you're lucky.'

Ronald nodded. 'That was one of my favourite parts of the retreat, the relaxation sessions with foot massage,' he said.

Maryliz held up a three-chambered clay vessel, the size and shape of an anatomical heart, and blew gently into the mouthpiece. Covering and uncovering the finger holes changed the pitch as her breath resonated inside the chambers, creating soft wind sounds with layers of overtones.

'Isn't the sound amazing, Marco? If I remember

correctly, Maryliz, the ocarina is a modern version of an ancient clay instrument from South America, right?' Ronald said, with his eyes closed. 'Marco, honey, you could lie beside me?' He patted the bed beside him.

Marco slid in beside Ronald, under the duvet.

I tiptoed to the end of the bed and untucked the duvet to expose Ronald's stockinged feet. I placed my hands under his soles and held them for a few moments before I began to stroke his feet, one at a time. Maryliz stood by Ronald's head and raised the ocarina to her lips.

The wind sounds seemed to cocoon the four of us in a protected space, safe against the march of time. I moved the palms of my hands in a downward motion from Ronald's ankles to the tips of his toes. Ronald's breath slowed into a steady rhythm, the in-breath and the out-breath of equal length, as though matching the waves of sound, coming and going. His eyelids twitched as he dropped into sleep.

I glanced at Marco, whose head rested in the crook of his bent right elbow while his other arm lay across Ronald's chest. The demands of caregiving were evident in Marco's pale worn face, but a life of loving lingered in their embrace as the breathy sounds of the ocarina wafted over us all.

16

HEATHER: The Plunge

H eather rented a yellow Volkswagen beetle for the trip to the weeklong cancer retreat, a car she had always coveted and never bought for herself. She couldn't justify a new car after her second diagnosis. She thought it would be a waste of money. After a five-hour flight from Toronto to Vancouver, and an hour-and-a-half ferry ride to Vancouver Island, she drove three hours across the mountains to Tofino, a small surfing town on the Pacific coast. Heather hoped the retreat would help her find peace, having been told by her oncologist that she had little time left to live. Being a doctor herself, she understood her grim prognosis from widespread metastases secondary to breast cancer.

Heather stepped out of the car at the front door of the lodge. Her wispy blonde hair, thinned from months on chemotherapy, was carefully tucked behind her ears and her tired grey eyes told the story of her long journey: the arduous road trip on that particular cold rainy day in mid-January, and the struggles of the past two years.

'Where's the beach, and my ocean?' she asked.

Heather had always wanted to visit the west coast, but given her busy medical practice, and the fact that her two kids played competitive sports in high school, there wasn't much time for family vacations, let alone a solo pilgrimage. I pointed to the narrow trailhead flanked by deer fern which wound steeply downhill to a sandy beach.

'I can hear her,' Heather said about the low, inter-mittent rumble of waves crashing on the beach below. The winter surf was high.

'Perhaps it would be best to wait until morning,' I suggested. 'Finding your way back up the trail in the dark might be tough, even with a flashlight.' I was concerned about Heather's compromised lungs for the climb back. 'Come on in and meet everyone. Dinner is almost ready.'

The smell of roast chicken greeted us as I pushed open the heavy wooden door into the lounge, with its floor-to-ceiling wood-burning fireplace, over-stuffed couches and picture windows on three sides of the room, overlooking the ocean.

After breakfast the next morning, I glanced out of the window and noticed four people on the beach far below and wondered if they were guests from the hotel nearby. Looking closer, I recognised Heather, and then Maria, followed by Susan and Betty. Despite the long days of travel, all four women had stayed up late the previous night, talking like old friends. They had much in common, including advanced cancer.

Two of the women wore bathing suits, one had on leggings and a sports top, and the fourth looked fully clothed other than her bare feet. It dawned on me slowly that four women with end-stage cancer, aged forty-two to fifty-five, were about to plunge into the white-capped waves of the Pacific Ocean in the middle of January. Holding hands, the tiny cluster of women then began to run slowly down the wet sand towards the steely grey-black sea.

I quickly gathered up a few other staff members, including Daphne, our retreat physician. We grabbed a stack of towels and rushed down the path to the beach. Off in the distance we could see four tiny heads appearing and disappearing between the waves of rolling surf. As we got closer to the water's edge, we saw bobbing smiles and heard high-pitched squeals above the sound of the surf. After a few minutes, one by one, the women found solid sand beneath their feet, stood up shakily, and waded their shivering bodies slowly through the surf and back onto the beach.

'If you can tame your fear of that freezing wild ocean, you can face anything at all,' Heather said, looking back over her shoulder at the sea. 'I didn't know until now, but I travelled almost five thousand kilometres to do that.'

She laughed as she held her cold wet palm to my cheek.

'Not going in?' she asked.

'Not on your life,' I said, then became suddenly aware of my faux pas.

Witnessing four women who knew they would die soon immerse themselves in the vast winter sea changed me in some indescribable way. Since that day in 1998, and as the promise of my body's impermanence settles in me, I remember those women and I say *Yes* more often to a whim, and surprise myself by overcoming a fear with courage. During the brief moments when I wondered if the women might perish in the freezing cold of the plunge that day, it also struck me that those minutes of gleeful abandon to the ocean might possibly have been worth the risk of an untimely end.

Heather died ten weeks after the retreat, and I always wondered if her wholehearted surrender to the ocean that day helped her in her last moments, to let go with courage into the vast unknown we know as death.

17

BILL: Thirteen Weeks

Bright yellow gorse, with its coconut fragrance, lined the footpath as we pushed against the wind. He wore his old black anorak, tweed cap and wellington boots smeared with mud from the garden. As we did most times I went home, Dad and I had hiked the five miles over the cliff to Sandyhills, in the southwest corner of Scotland, pausing at Castle Point for a few minutes to catch our breath and to follow the arrows carved in the stone marker with our eyes, out into the steel-grey sea towards Canada, my home of the past twelve years. Everyone said that Dad and I were 'two of a kind'. We'd always had a relationship that didn't depend on words. We knew how the other one felt without needing to talk about it. And that day in 1996, just after his sixty-seventh birthday, was no different.

Three months after that hike, Dad was diagnosed with a Stage IV brain tumour. He called me to come home the day after he got the news. Perhaps he felt that I would know what to do, since I had worked as an oncology nurse for fifteen years by then. However, for me, my career dissolved during that phone conversation. I was a daughter, not a nurse then, and working with other people with cancer while my father was dying made no sense. I took leave and planned a trip to Scotland, where I'd spend most of the next thirteen weeks of my father's illness.

Sudden memory loss had taken him to his family doctor. The scan showed a large inoperable brain tumour. His oncologist said treating a glioblastoma was futile, that the side effects would strip him of dignity for the time he had left. No surgery, chemotherapy or radiation meant a sure death, but also the hope of a dignified one.

'I have a brain tumour, deep-seated, in the centre of my brain? Is that right?' he asked me over dinner, the first evening I arrived.

'You do, Dad. It's a Stage IV brain tumour called a glioblastoma.'

'I have a deep-seated brain tumour, don't I? Will it kill me?' His short-term memory loss made it hard for him to retain information.

'Yes, it will, Dad. I'm so sorry. The oncologist

told you at your first appointment that you'll probably only live three or four months.' My voice quivered.

'What do I have – a deep-seated tumour in my brain? Is it malignant?' he asked again.

My father, a brilliant, educated man who had received a knighthood from Prince Philip for his work in the arts, couldn't retain one fact.

At first my answers were soft and careful. I couldn't pretend, as I'd heard many do, and attach false hope to my responses. He asked again and again, trying to hold on to the tragedy that kept dissolving in his mind. Impatience slowly crept in on the heels of my waning tolerance to his repetitive questions.

'Dad, you have cancer, and you are going to die in three to four months.' My voice was short and clipped, almost hostile.

Truth must have landed with a thud into a part of his brain that still functioned when he responded, 'I'm going to die? Well, then, no monks' urine for me. That's what people do, don't they, when they get cancer? They travel around the world looking for cures. I'm not that kind of man. I've had a good life, and I'll just get going out of here. It'll be harder on your mum.' He looked at me and I saw the sadness of leaving in his eyes.

He spent only one night of the next thirteen weeks in hospital. We checked him into the neurosurgery ward to have the brain biopsy that would confirm what the brain scan showed. I was relieved that the diagnosis wouldn't be made purely on the basis of technology; the biopsy would ensure that the cancer was seen with the naked eye.

The nurse showed us to his bed, one of ten lined up side-by-side against one wall in a nineteenth-century Nightingale-style ward, with ten more on the opposite wall. The tiny nursing station was perched in the middle of the extra-shiny linoleum floor which I knew from experience the nurses shined up on the weekend with an electric polisher. Every patient's health report was discussed aloud by a group of ten to twelve doctors who stood around each bed every morning before first light. I knew Dad's brain status would be known by many other patients the next morning before he was rolled off to the operating room. That felt oddly comforting. I hoped they would send him good thoughts while he was under the knife.

Mum pulled the flimsy orange curtain around the bed in her attempt to create a private world for the three of us. I could hear the low hum of chatter from other patients' visitors, and if anyone could, they would understand our pain.

Dad looked older and smaller in the pale blue hospital pyjamas with a button missing midway down. He perched on top of crisp white sheets over a plastic-covered mattress which crinkled every time he moved. He had kept his socks on. Bare feet against the cold sheets was too much vulnerability perhaps.

After an hour or so, Mum and I bid a hasty farewell, guilty in our abandonment.

'See you tomorrow, darling,' she whispered, and kissed Dad lightly on the lips.

Losing your mind is not all bad. Dad lost his future as well as his past, and death lives in the future. His worries had taken a back seat and he was softer, more at ease. Without his memory, he also lost the roles and identities that defined his life. Dad was a husband and father, a successful businessman, and a golfer. He was an introvert, with a dry sense of humour. He loved the six of us playing his made-up general knowledge quizzes after Sunday dinners.

'What is the capital of Iceland? Now spell it.'

'What is the meaning of the word *taciturn*?' he'd ask. My two sisters, brother and I would shake our heads. 'Nancy, what about you?'

Mum always squirmed when she didn't know the answer.

'Quiet and withdrawn,' he'd say. 'Like me.'

He dragged the family off on many bitterly cold weekends to look at lighthouses for sale. He'd talk a boatman into ferrying us across rough sea to some tiny barren island, and to pick us up a few hours later, frozen and miserable. He fancied the life of a hermit, but then would joke about having to put up with all of us. He never did buy a lighthouse.

He was loyal and kind, irritable and particular. He loved the poems of John Donne and read books about the Second World War. I relied on him in ways I only understood after he was gone. My human encyclopedia was missing. My lazy method of research had always been to pick up the phone and ask him any historical or political question, and he'd always known the answer. He'd studied medieval history at university. I also hadn't known that his presence on the planet made me feel safe in the world until he died.

We sent the nurse home earlier than usual the night Dad died. My two sisters and I felt uncomfortable sitting across the room from a relative stranger in the intimate space that my parents had shared for thirty-eight years.

Most people's breathing slows down at the end of life, but my father's sped up. He sounded like he was working hard. His eyelids were closed and the skin on his face looked as youthful as his soft brown hair, not yet grey. As a kid, I remember rubbing the palm of my hand against his close-shaven chin, and giggling at the roughness of it. There was something about his maleness that intrigued me.

Mum sat close, her hand in his. Every few moments she stroked his face or his hair, and said, 'It's okay, Bill.'

Even with the imminent separation from her beloved, she seemed to know that death was merciful. The creases of worry in her face were softer. Death wasn't frightening. It was natural. A wife, three daughters and a daughter-in-law were accompanying a great man out of this world.

It surprised us when his eyes suddenly opened wide. The green was brighter than I had remembered. He looked directly at my mother, and she was there to receive him. Those seconds would last for ever as I felt the depth of thirty-eight years pass between them. Love like that had no need for words.

Then his last breath. In or out, I don't know. No petering out, though. Just the one breath, and then the great silence that fell upon us.

Mum wanted to sleep in the room beside him, to have one last night in the presence of her husband's body, although it was mottled and cold by then. She didn't sleep much, and I imagined her reminiscing all night about the years she spent getting to know every inch of his body with her touch. At first light she washed him and dressed him in a pair of clean, carefully ironed pyjamas.

I was given pocket money to iron his clothes as a kid. The large cotton handkerchiefs were my favourite, ironed and folded in a particular way to flick perfectly out of his top jacket pocket. The pyjamas were always the most difficult, trying to smooth all the creases, flipping them back and forth on the ironing board.

Mum was a nurse too, so she knew the skilful way to dress someone in bed after they've died. You roll them towards you, propping a pillow in behind to keep them from falling back. A second person is helpful, but Mum wanted to do it alone.

Around mid-morning, she nodded with an air of quiet resignation. Soon we heard the scrunch of the hearse on the gravel outside. Two solemn men came to the door; one carried a collapsible stretcher under his arm. They looked like they were on an errand to pick up something that needed returning to the store. If they'd smiled, even slightly, it might have helped. Death feels sad, not indifferent.

My sister Kate stayed with Mum in the living room while I showed the funeral directors into the bedroom. I hoped they would move him with respect. I didn't want to watch, in case they didn't. Some bodies are moved from hospital beds as though they are furniture. I always want to say, 'Be careful, please, he belongs to a family.'

They wheeled Dad out of the front door, feet first. Mum had been adamant about not watching him being taken from the house, but I saw her standing bereft behind the glass of the living-room door. The holding on, and the letting go, all wrapped up in that one glance.

I remember the empty feeling then, the deep ache of never going back. I'd never have another father.

Snow had fallen that December morning, as if to echo our inner coldness. The pale winter sunshine pressed itself through the bare branches of the great silver birch at the top of the driveway, calling me outside. There wasn't much snow to shovel but it was a good excuse to remind myself that life was still moving through the bones and muscles of my body.

The driveway from the gate down to the garage door was steep, and I knew Mum would insist on shovelling the snow herself if I didn't get to it first. She'd likely walk up to the shops the next morning, as she did every morning, to fetch the *Herald*. I didn't want her to slip and break any limbs. In her grief, she'd be preoccupied and unaware of her footsteps around the potholes and puddles on Horseshoe Road.

Opening the garage door from the inside, I stepped out and felt the biting cold penetrate the fog in my brain. I hadn't been out of the house for three days. A surprising lightness lifted my spirits as I shovelled mounds of powdery snow off the driveway. It was satisfying to be engaged in a solvable problem. For thirteen weeks we had been locked into an unfixable situation with no solution, only a sure ending.

A flicker of red caught my eye. I heard the first notes of her song before I saw her. The tiny robin, with her bright breast, was perched on a low branch of a frosty azalea about three feet from my left boot. Her glossy black eyes seemed to take me in as she chirped her melody. Her trills of seven high notes of different pitches repeated like a mantra, and I felt her carry me away to a place where delight still lived.

The robin then hopped off her branch and flew directly into the open door of the garage. Landing first on the roof of Dad's car, she looked around to contemplate her route. From his golf clubs, she took off from the putter and hopped along the row of gardening tools to his big, muddy wellington boots. I remembered climbing into his boots as a child, shoes and all, and shuffling along the garden path.

Touching down briefly onto his tweed cap, the robin then took her leave. I watched her swoop low to clear the retracted garage door and fly up over the back gate until she disappeared into the sky.

18

JEN: Awe

I was one of the lucky ones who received regular Wicky email updates from Jen, a past retreat participant and later a volunteer and board member. She had befriended a hummingbird she nicknamed after her favourite place on the planet, the Wickaninnish Inn in Tofino. She and her husband Gerald and their dog Berlo tried to get out to the wild Pacific coast of Vancouver Island every year for vacations. Jen shared with those of us on her email list her surprise at seeing a hummingbird on Chesterman Beach, near the inn, in blustery west-coast weather, and had thought about how robust the little bird was to survive.

Jen felt anything but robust when she first met the hummingbird she named Wicky on her deck at home. She was recuperating from brain radiation for metastases, secondary to breast cancer. I met her first when she attended a Callanish retreat two years before the recurrence of cancer, and we had stayed in touch. I learned this story of her connection to this little bird and was so moved by the inspiration that nature offers, often at the times we need it most.

Out of the corner of one eye Jen noticed a flash of iridescent green amidst the new bamboo shoots emerging from shiny black stems. She had planted a pot of black bamboo two years before, on the small patio adjacent to the sliding glass door of her home office. She loved the way the wind rustled through the tall stems and new leaves in the spring, casting light and shadow across her work surface.

She saw the green flash again as a rufous humming-bird flew into the bamboo with strands of dried moss dangling from its tiny beak. The nest was miraculously attached to one of the wider stems of bamboo, just a few inches from the glass door. Jen was mesmerised as the hummingbird returned again and again, bringing pieces of light grey lichen, shavings of wood, and fine silver threads from spider webs. The tiny construction project was well under way by the time Jen succumbed an hour later to her daily afternoon nap.

When she had awakened earlier that morning, she'd been overcome by the desire to pull the covers over her head and retreat from the world. She had promised her husband Gerald, as he leaned over to kiss her goodbye, that she would get out of bed, make breakfast, and attempt to get some work done at her desk downstairs.

'Don't waste the day,' he called to her from the stairs on the way to the garage.

Easy for you to say, she thought to herself. *You try being chipper when you've just had your brain irradiated five days in a row.* She'd been annoyed with him for days. In fact, she was angry with every healthy person she encountered. Her family and friends had no idea what it was like, at forty, to be dealing with a second recurrence of breast cancer in just six years. Most of her friends were wrapped up in successful careers and looking after young children, too busy to spend time with her. An occasional text or email was the best they could do. She understood their priorities, but was still hurt by their neglect.

'Don't worry, honey. Have a good day,' she had called back.

Her oncologist said it would take at least six weeks of rest to regain her energy. She worried that she'd lose her mind from the radiation, although her oncologist assured her she wouldn't. She had entered the deep, dark landscape of depression, a state she had only felt once before, when she had been told her cancer had spread to her bones.

In her early twenties Jen was a ski model in Switzerland, participating in extreme ski films, and later became a sports clothing designer after moving back to Canada for school. Since her re-diagnosis, Jen could barely walk around the block and could only keep up with small design projects. She created an office at home for the days she felt like tackling work. Feeling purposeful kept the foreboding at bay.

The morning after the hummingbird's arrival, Jen woke up with a lift in her mood. She didn't linger long in bed after Gerald left for work. With a cup of good strong coffee in hand, she made her way down to her office to check on the nest. She settled into the big armchair, wrapped a blanket around her knees, and waited. Sure enough, mid-morning, the hummingbird returned, flying in and out of the bamboo with dried leaf threads and strands of wood mulch. She counted thirty-two trips in one hour. The hummingbird glued the pieces together with spiders' webs by burrowing against the sides of the nest, spreading the sticky threads with her breast and hopping up and down to shape the floor. The hummingbird worked for four hours that day and Jen spent most of that time tucked into her own nest, thoroughly engaged in every step of the building process.

'How did your day go, sweetheart?' Gerald asked as he pulled off his blazer and tie. Jen lay on the bed reading about hummingbirds on her iPad. She felt guilty that it was dinner time and she was too fatigued to stand in the kitchen and prepare food, as she often had before cancer.

'Not bad,' she said. 'Didn't get any work done, mind you.'

'How come?'

'Wicky kept me entertained,' she said.

'Who?'

'Wicky, our resident hummingbird. She's building a nest in the bamboo downstairs, can you believe it?' Jen was excited, a feeling she hadn't felt for many weeks.

She escorted him downstairs to show him the nest. Wicky had left for the day and Jen wondered where she slept at night, imagining her collapsed in a pile of leaves after a hard day's work. She felt as if she was showing Gerald something she had made herself, like when she used to present a new design, hesitant and hoping for his approval. She felt proud of Wicky's industriousness and handiwork. She imagined that preparing for birth would require a lot of stamina.

Jen had never wanted children; neither had Gerald. She was sure cancer had something to do with their decision, given that she'd been diagnosed at such a young age, but they hadn't talked about it much. Too risky perhaps, the thought of getting sick again and leaving their children without a mother, like her mother had when Jen was eleven years old. Being a motherless daughter had been difficult, empty and confusing during all of her teenage years, and she hadn't understood much about her mother's cancer and why she died so quickly over just a few weeks. Besides, she and Gerald loved the life they had together without children. They thought of each other as soulmates.

Five days after the first sighting, Wicky spent more and more time sitting in her nest. She looked comical squished into the tiny woven cup, with her wing feathers fluffing out over the rim and long tail feathers standing upright. Wicky's eyes flickered from side to side constantly, as though scanning for threats, and occasionally her eyes would close for a few moments.

Each morning thereafter, Jen woke earlier than usual. She looked forward to spending the day in her big armchair downstairs and hardly noticed her tiredness or vague, persistent headache. On the morning of Day 7, Jen saw that Wicky was gone, so she carefully positioned a footstool against the glass, stepped up and looked down into the tiny nest. She saw two minuscule white eggs, the size of marbles, lying side by side. She felt a surge of love push through the glass from her heart at these miracles of creation, and the thought of the tiny heartbeats already fluttering inside.

Jen and Wicky sat nestled in, day after day, keeping one another company in the waiting. Jen rarely thought about her illness. Caring about another living being had swept her up, distracted her from her problems. Awe had become the antidote to despair.

Wicky left the nest for about ten minutes every hour, so Jen would take the opportunity to look inside and snap photographs. She sent the pictures along with 'Wicky Updates' by email to her family and friends, and they responded with great interest. She began to feel connected to the outside world again. Every evening when Gerald got home, they had their pre-dinner glass of wine together in her office downstairs while Jen described Wicky's day. She wasn't as annoyed with Gerald any more because she had news to contribute to their evening conversation. For months she had had nothing fresh to bring to their relationship, or to her friendships, except complaints about symptoms and fears for her future.

On windy nights, Jen worried about Wicky swaying back and forth in her nest, on her mini rollercoaster. She had to develop faith that Wicky knew what she was doing by choosing the location of her babies' home, tucked into the stems of the bamboo.

At Day 20 since the start of the nest-building, Jen noticed Wicky was perched on the side of the nest looking in. She left the nest for only a few minutes at a time for food, and on one of those forays Jen looked into the nest from her footstool and saw two tiny, brown, featherless, squirming shapes with open mouths. The eggs had hatched and Wicky had three weeks to feed them with pollen and tiny insects, regurgitated into the babies' mouths, until they were strong enough to learn to fly. A week or so later, Jen noticed the first feathers, and after another week the babies filled out the nest almost to breaking point. At Day 40, the baby hummingbirds made their first flight under the watchful eye of Jen, and for the next two days Wicky and her two babies took longer and longer flights away from the nest. On Day 43, six weeks and one day from the start of the nest-building, the baby hummingbirds were gone.

In the weeks that followed, Jen would occasionally spot one of the fledglings at her feeder and her heart would flip with joy. Jen had become so engrossed in the cycle of new life throughout her six-week recuperation that she barely noticed her strength returning, and the hair beginning to grow back on her once-bald head.

19

KATE: The Dance

I had never seen a dying woman dance before. Her large belly full of cancer and her laboured breathing didn't seem to impede the ease and grace with which she swayed to the rhythms of the Cuban music. I imagined her hair before the chemotherapy: dark, thick and shiny, turning this way and that as she tossed her head in time to the congas. But Kate's hair was about an inch long. Rebellious dark spikes pushed out as if to say, *You can't keep me down for long.* It felt to me as though Kate had been put on earth for that moment, to dance then and there for us, for herself, and for her life. None of us had known Kate was a professional salsa dancer until she took to the floor on that last day of the retreat.

I had met Kate in my counselling office a few

months before. Her world had collapsed. She knew pancreatic cancer was usually a death sentence.

'She won't remember me, will she?' Kate whispered, referring to her three-year-old daughter, Polly.

I knew the answer she hoped for by the expression of longing and trepidation in her deep brown eyes, but Kate pre-empted my response with more questions. 'Do you know other little girls who have lost their moms?' she asked. 'How have they done in their lives without a mommy?'

I told her about Natasha.

Peter was a client of mine who'd brought his nine-year-old daughter Natasha for the first of several counselling sessions. His wife Elaine had seen me in her final stages of cancer, and she'd made him promise to bring Natasha for bereavement support. But six years had passed and Peter never came. He felt Natasha was coping okay without her mom. However, when their family dog died, Natasha was inconsolable, and Peter finally called for an appointment.

Natasha was slight in build and tall for a nine-year-old. Her shoulder-length, wavy blonde hair hung free, which conveyed a kind of self-confidence. She met my gaze at the door and said 'Hello' in a curious manner.

'Do you feel okay to come with me for a chat by

yourself, or would you prefer it if your dad came with us?' I asked.

'I'm okay.' She looked to her dad for approval, and he nodded.

Natasha and I walked around the Callanish centre and I acquainted her with the different therapy rooms. First, the art studio with its paints, papers, collage images, clay and fabrics. I watched her face light up as she looked around.

'I like this room,' she said.

'I met you when you were two years old, when your mom brought you here a few times after she first got sick. You loved this room then, especially when you got to do body-painting and make a big mess. I'm sad she's not here today with you and I'm really, really sad she died.'

I wanted her to know I was aware of her mom's death and that it was okay to talk about it if she wanted to.

'Yup, me too,' Natasha said, and changed the subject. 'Do you have to use water for these paints? The ones I have at home don't need water.'

'These paints don't need water,' I said.

We continued the tour of the building and I showed Natasha the sandtray room, with its multiple shelves from floor to ceiling filled with small objects: people, animals, feathers, stones, shells, toys, miniature houses and furniture, fairies and wizards, religious and secular symbols, as well as medical and hospital items like syringes and pill bottles. The sandtray room helps children and adults talk about difficult subjects that can be more easily expressed by creating stories, using objects placed in a tray of sand.

'Can I make a picture in the sand?' Natasha asked.

'Sure,' I said and handed her a small basket, suggesting she choose objects she liked, as well as some she didn't like, as many as she wanted. The unconscious mind attaches to objects that have a positive or negative association, and can evoke helpful insights into a predicament. I pointed to the stepladder for Natasha to reach the top shelves. She looked carefully at every shelf and chose about thirty objects, climbing to the top shelves to be thorough in her exploration before placing them in the basket.

After she finished, I pointed to the large wooden sandtray filled with fine golden sand. 'You can put the objects in the sand any way you want. You'll sense where you want to put them. Take your time.'

Natasha was quiet as she carefully placed her objects in a pattern that made no apparent sense to me, but was clearly deliberate and considered.

'Would you tell me the story?' I asked when she was finished.

Natasha told me about her family. She chose figurines for her father, her three brothers, her four grandparents, her cousins, aunts and uncles, and her three best friends at school. She also chose pieces for her dance teacher and her best friend's mom. As she pointed to each figurine in the tray, she told me their names, their ages, and a story about each person. She chose an eagle for her mother and balanced it on the one-inch ledge of the wooden sandtray. She also added a few houses, trees, a miniature bonfire, a guitar, some shells, and a mirror to represent water.

'My favourite times with my family are when we all go to Salt Spring Island for family reunions. We stay in six different cabins and have bonfires on the beach every night and sing songs.' Her face was bright as she remembered.

'Your mom would have loved to be there, don't you think?' I suggested.

'She'd have loved it. Dad told me she liked to sing. She even sang in a choir and made a CD once. We play it at home lots.' Natasha was animated as she told me her family stories. 'I chose an eagle for Mom because she loved eagles. She is looking down at everyone and is happy we are having fun,' she said.

'What is it like not having a mom?' I asked Natasha.

'I'm kinda used to it. The worst time is at school when they talk about Mother's Day and make stuff, and I feel weird,' she said.

'That must be hard. What do you do?' I asked.

'I make a card for my grandma,' Natasha said. 'She's my mom's mom. She has told me so many stories about my mom that I feel like I know her. Everyone says I'm just like her.' She smiled.

'What about your dog?' I asked. 'Do you want to put him in the sandtray story?'

One large single tear rolled down Natasha's cheek and dropped onto the sand.

'He died,' she said.

'Your dad told me. I'm so sorry,' I said. 'You must miss him.'

Natasha sniffed loudly. 'I miss him so much. He's been with me my whole life. He always slept in my bed with me.'

I asked her if she wanted to choose an object to represent her dog so he could still be part of the family. She considered carefully, picking up each of the dog figurines and turning them over in her hands until she selected one. 'Rupert wasn't exactly like this dog, but a bit like it.'

She walked over to the sandtray and balanced the dog beside the eagle on the ledge. She sat quietly and looked at both objects for a long time.

'I wish they were here,' she said. 'But at least they're together, and they can see us, and know we're having fun.'

* * *

Kate had nodded her head continuously through my story, as though acknowledging the truth of it, that Polly would soon have to find ways to accept her mom's death like Natasha did.

'Will you help Polly when she gets older?' she asked.

'Of course I will.'

A couple of months after that counselling session, Kate attended a weeklong Callanish retreat. She wanted to learn how to accept her dying, in the hope that she could then help her daughter find a way through the pain of loss.

One morning during the group session, Kate began to articulate her fears for her daughter. 'I don't think I can bear it, imagining Polly living without me and me not being there for her,' she said. Her hands were shaking.

The room was quiet for a few moments until all of a sudden Kate screamed. The agony rose from the depths of her maternal soul, piercing the illusion of any guarantee of life's fairness or certainty. Wave after wave of grief and despair washed through her as sobs wracked her body. I moved my chair closer to her. Time seemed to stand still as the group waited, submerged in the archetypal pain of all mothers who grieve separation from their children too soon. The group's faith in Kate's ability to withstand her agony would be her medicine.

After what seemed like a very long time, the wailing stopped. A deep calm pervaded the room and the silence lingered. Kate's pain had been dispersed into a community of people who were able to tolerate its expression because they too lived with anguish.

Finally, Kate cast her eyes around the group, acknowledging each person's companionship on her journey to the deep. She had arrived back onto new ground after surrendering to extreme vulnerability.

Two days later, in the closing circle of the retreat, Kate spoke up.

'I would like to thank you all, by way of this dance, for the strength you've offered me, to hear and care about my pain.'

The group members pushed their chairs to the edges of the room, clearing a space in the centre of the room for the dance.

When the Cuban music began, Kate pushed herself to standing, using both armrests of her chair. She walked slowly into the centre of the room and paused. Her eyes looked up as though trying to reach for something familiar, perhaps connecting to a lineage of salsa dancers who understood that the dance can enliven the spirit and lift a person out of the challenges of daily life. Kate began to move in slow, small steps in time to the guitar and drums, raising her arms above her head in short rhythmic gestures around her erect spine and neck. Kate seemed enraptured by an energy that took her body into faster and faster movements as the pace of the music quickened. She swirled and twirled in time to the beat. After about ten minutes, the music stopped and all we could hear was her rapid jagged breathing which pierced the silence. Kate closed her eyes for a few moments, as if savouring the life force that was moving through her ailing body. When she finally looked around the room into captivated faces, her eyes blazed with light.

When Kate took to the dance floor that day, it appeared that she had plunged into an aspect of herself that was living, not dying. I sensed that she had been able to locate this place because of her surrender into the pain of her imminent loss, bringing her into a deep connection to her suffering. As Kate swirled around the room, oblivious to the rapt faces of the people around her, she was perhaps carried away by the music to a place where there was no cancer or dying, no large belly or shortness of breath, a place where her spirit could be free.

During the eight weeks after that retreat Kate dedicated most of her time to creating a legacy for her daughter. She asked her husband to conduct a series of video interviews with her, explaining the story of Polly's birth, and the feelings she had had when she first held Polly, and her adventures learning to be a mom to a daughter she couldn't believe she could love so much. She audiotaped herself reading Polly's favourite stories and singing her most-loved nursery rhymes. She reassured Polly that no matter what happened in her life, she would always be with her in some way. She wanted Polly to know always how much she had loved her.

I believe the work Kate did at the retreat to face the reality of her dying, coming into direct contact with her pain, helped her to complete this legacy work for her daughter. Without the work and the support of the group, Kate would likely not have had the stamina to do what for many dying people feels insurmountable.

Kate was admitted to hospice a few months later, and Polly came to visit with her dad a few times. Like Natasha, Polly is blessed with an extended family that is committed to keeping the stories of her mom alive. I still see both girls from time to time for counselling, and although the pain of their losses continues to surface after more than fifteen years, they both lead meaningful and productive lives. Natasha is now a mother of two beautiful little girls.

20

LIZ: Excruciating Beauty

Doug stepped towards me and held out the black plastic box of his wife's cremated remains. 'Take a handful if you'd like to,' he said, his eyebrows raised in the hopes that I would. I tried to imagine being as generous with my beloved's ashes. I think I'd want to keep them all for myself and not want to share, not want to let go, not want to be so inclusive.

My breath quickened at the thought of touching my dear friend Liz's ashes with my bare hands. It felt so intimate somehow. But I pushed my hand into the darkness of the box anyway and allowed myself to feel Liz's once-animated body coat my fingers in cool, dense, bony ash. I paused briefly before closing my fist around some part of her and lifting her out of the box. I wanted to take my time then, to look at the ashes up close, to smell them, to let them run through my fingers like I did as a kid with the sand on the beach at Southend for hours on end, wondering about the eons of time that had passed to turn stone into deep yellow sand. I was curious to examine the transmutation of a body by fire, to know this Liz, to know what my body will become too one day. But I felt the nudge to keep moving, so with barely a glance into the grey ash I cupped my left hand protectively over my right, keeping it safe, keeping *her* safe, in the dark warmth of my cradled hands.

When we had designed the ceremony a week before, Doug knew he wanted to spread some of Liz's ashes on top of the flower mandala we would create as a community. The year before, I had watched Tibetan monks for hours as they created a sand mandala at the Museum of Anthropology among the vast totem poles of the Pacific Northwest Coast First Nations, and was captivated by the intricacy, the precise patterns and the quiet with which the monks created their representation of consciousness. After five days, the monks ceremonially swept their creation into a mound of multi-coloured sand and carried it in procession to the ocean, where they chanted prayers before releasing it into the water. Nothing is permanent; all is impermanent; a thought I want to fiercely reject when it comes to the people I love.

What Doug didn't know until the ceremony had begun was that he would also want to invite others to sprinkle some of Liz's ashes onto the reds, oranges, yellows and whites of rose petals, lilies and gerberas placed by loved ones onto a large white canvas circle on the floor.

In the three years since Liz's son and daughter had left for university, she had delved into her creative life: learning to make burrata and chocolate, writing poems, painting abstracts with bright acrylics, sewing cushion covers for the arts and crafts furniture Doug had made for their living room. Liz deeply understood the role of beauty in her own healing, and for all the people with cancer we had cared for together in our work of the past ten years. The flower mandala we would create for Liz that day seemed like a fitting tribute.

After fifty people had carefully arranged the petals collected from their gardens, or from the retreat centre grounds, onto the mandala, Doug first offered the box of ashes to his son Will, and then to his daughter Jacqueline. I felt my heart push out of my chest towards them, to comfort them, to salve their pain, but then I noticed that I felt strangely reassured by their willingness, their capacity to come into direct contact with this tangible and radically altered form of mother – but mother nonetheless – to touch her and grace her and offer her up to the bed of beauty at our feet. I felt the love and support of community close in on them as others mirrored their courage to step forward.

I was brought back to my own father's cremation, exactly twenty years before. I sat in a cold, grey, life-less room in a crematorium in Glasgow with about twenty family members, all of us dressed in black, while we watched my father's coffin get transferred mechanically from the raised platform a few feet in front of us, through a set of grey shiny acrylic curtains, the kind you'd see in a cheap motel room except these ones were opened and closed by an invisible operator. Nothing was said, no music was played, there was no colour and no beauty. We were passive observers to an impersonal and mysterious process of how Dad's body would be turned to ashes.

Kneeling on the floor beside the flower mandala, I brought my cupped hands to my lips and kissed my gratitude to Liz through my living skin and bones and blood. Praying for her release into beauty, I sprinkled the ashes over the orange and red rose petals and yellow lilies, and watched as the bright colours faded to grey. I was deeply aware of my friends kneeling around the circle too, being as close to our beloved Liz as we could possibly be in her absence.

Liz was my right-hand person at work, who made my life easier and better – an expert in organisational flow and systems. She was also a woman who deeply understood the sorrow and fear and utter devastation of a diagnosis, and the potential for hope and healing garnered from thirty-three years of her own lived experience of cancer. I relied on her in ways I only understood once she left work, suddenly, after a third diagnosis of cancer.

Liz and I first met when she came to one of our weeklong cancer retreats as a participant, after her second breast cancer diagnosis, eighteen years after her first diagnosis at the age of twenty-nine. Liz told me that her primary reason for coming on retreat was to grieve the loss of her mother, who had died at the age of forty-nine when Liz was eighteen. As the eldest of three, Liz had had to put her sorrow away to take on the responsibility for helping her dad manage the household. She hadn't known what else to do. With her second diagnosis in her late forties, around the age that her mom died, Liz's grief had caught up with her and she needed a safe place to tend to it.

She cried more than she talked that week on retreat, and by the last day she told me how good it felt to finally let her heart break open, to feel the sorrow she had carried unattended for eighteen years. Liz stayed connected to Callanish over the next five years, attending the monthly support group for past retreat participants and volunteering in the office when she could, between her work of managing a family business and looking after her two teenaged children. When the office manager job opened up at Callanish, she was the obvious choice.

I first heard Liz's shallow cough one morning in the office we shared every day. Being an oncology nurse, I notice coughs and quickly assess them: dry, productive, deep, shallow, persistent, wheezy, hacking, worrisome, not worrisome. I listened to her coughing for a couple of weeks before I asked her if she had had it checked out. She told me she had been to see her family doctor and was on antibiotics, so I relaxed – somewhat. Meanwhile, we carried on each day, welcoming people with cancer into our centre for support.

About a month later, Liz was driving into work when she suddenly noticed a numbness spreading down her right arm and across her chest. She drove herself straight to the emergency room. The CT scan showed a mass in the top lobe of her right lung that the doctor told her was likely cancer. She would need a biopsy to know the exact pathology.

Liz was now sixty-one and it was looking like a third cancer diagnosis, which I assumed would be metastatic spread to her lung from the original breast cancer. I knew many women with metastatic breast cancer who were living well and I drew hope from their stories in my mind as I tried to grapple with Liz's horrible news.

We left for our spring retreat a week after Liz's visit to Emergency. She had undergone a multitude of tests during that week, including a liver biopsy, but the numbness had resolved and she was feeling well enough to come on the retreat as a cook, as she had done for ten years, every season. Engaging in purposeful work while waiting for the test results would be a good distraction.

On the last day of the retreat the call came from Doug on my cellphone. Liz had told me that she didn't want to recieve any calls from her doctors while on retreat and that she had asked Doug to take any urgent calls on her behalf.

'Janie, it's not good,' he said.

A chill ran up my spine. I remembered how Mum used to say when I was a kid that a shiver up my spine was someone walking over my grave. Bad news always hits my body first, before my mind and heart. Like when I received the phone call from my mother, out of the blue, to say my dad had a brain tumour, not the treatable kind, but a glioblastoma. The oncologist said it was 'game over'. My body shook for several minutes after I hung up the phone with her that day.

'Doug, you need to tell Liz first, before you tell me,' I said, cutting him off. I couldn't bear the thought of knowing something before she did, and I didn't want to be the one to break bad news to her. My thoughts flashed to all the oncologists I knew who had the harrowing task of telling people test results that would change their lives for ever. I grasped this mammoth undertaking in ways that I hadn't understood before.

'Can you tell her I will call in five minutes? And can you be with her when I call? It's not good,' Doug said again.

'I'm sorry, Doug, I really am.'

The news was worse than metastatic breast cancer. There are a lot more options for treating recurrent breast cancer than for a Stage IV lung cancer spread to the liver. Liz was not a candidate for surgery and would start immediate experimental chemotherapy. She didn't want to hear a prognosis, but given my experience I thought she would live for a year if she was lucky.

By contrast, my father *did* want to hear his prognosis. He asked the oncologist for it in his matter-of-fact way.

'How long have I got?'

'Three to four months,' the oncologist had said.

When Dad heard the prediction, I saw hope drop

to the floor before he had the chance to hold it in his hands. He trusted the scientists. He wasn't going to waste time wishing for a miracle or seeking out alternative therapies. He wanted to drink champagne and watch old episodes of his favourite television show, *Dad's Army*, and have quality time with his wife of thirty-eight years and his four kids when they could get home for a visit. But his kids, myself and my three siblings, unlike Liz's, had established lives, careers, spouses and children, independent from him. He had lived a satisfying life, one he could accept letting go of, albeit with a trough of sadness.

Unlike my father, Liz had lived in relationship with cancer for her entire adult life, and had been cured twice. Perhaps her enduring hope with this third diagnosis was based on her lived experience of a body that trusted chemotherapy to ensure a cure, and even with a Stage IV lung cancer diagnosis, with such grim statistics, her body memory of being twice cured could keep her hope alive. If Liz could control her mind and accompanying emotions by choosing not to have conversations about prognosis and inevitable death with her doctors and her friends, then life would likely hold more promise for however long she lived.

Liz lived the first ten months of her diagnosis with hope and determination.

'Why not, Janie? Some people defy the statistics – 1 per cent of people with Stage IV lung cancer survive past five years, and we know someone who has survived nine years, don't we?' Liz said, her gaze urging me to agree.

I did know Diana, who had received the same diagnosis, and she *was* living in the 1 per cent. I wanted so badly to hope alongside Liz, but a constant feeling of foreboding pressed into the pit of my stomach. I tried to will my mind to ignore that feeling because, after all, I had been wrong about Louise, another retreat participant. She had accused me of giving up hope. When she was taken off the palliative care programme for being too well, and then lived five years longer than predicted by her oncologist, I had to review my faulty prognosis. I *had* given up hope for Louise, so I knew that my predictions about life and death were not always reliable.

In the early months, I tried very hard to ignore the foreboding and wished and hoped alongside Liz that she could be one of the extraordinary ones who survived Stage IV lung cancer. When the chemotherapy took away the persistent cough and breathlessness, and the radiation helped her bone pain, it was easier to do. Liz even worked a few hours at the office, and I could forget the cancer for a few moments and believe we would work side-by-side until one of us finally decided to retire.

As the months went on, my hope waned. Liz's didn't. I think it was the nurse in me that saw the developing signs – weight loss, swollen ankles, declining energy, occasional mental confusion, and the yellow hue that filmed the whites of her eyes. I didn't want to see those things, but I did.

I even worried that my lack of hope might somehow have an effect on Liz's survival. A few nights before my father died, I questioned whether my peace with and acceptance of his dying might somehow prevent his chance for a miracle. I wanted to feel like the bystander I learned about in social psychology class who, when surrounded by other people in a crisis, would succumb to bystander apathy and believe that nothing was really wrong. I knew, though, that the deeper feeling I was having with my father, and with Liz, was that I didn't *want* them to be dying and that I was devastated. The magical thinking that I could somehow prevent a miracle or hasten death by my thinking was just my inability to accept that I had no control over what was happening.

Once I made space inside for my own helplessness, I could surrender to the truth of the situation and find some peace alongside my sorrow. My father surrendered to death right at the moment of his diagnosis, and Liz would hold tight to her life until there was no choice but to let go. There is clearly no right way.

'Until my oncologist tells me it's over, and there is no more treatment, then I will keep hoping,' Liz said. 'And I want you to hold the intention with me.'

The tension between us was palpable. My heart pounded. It felt like I was being asked to do the impossible.

'I will do my best, Lizzy, my friend,' I said, and took her hand in mine. 'You know I want you to be here, more than anything.' I saw the flicker of disappointment in her eyes as she registered my doubt in her miracle.

I realised then that I had an agenda that included talking about dying and the things that might be important to her in her last weeks. After all, Liz and I and our team had supported hundreds of people with cancer through their healing and their dying processes over the past decade. I knew that those types of conversations would dissolve the tension for me, and bring us closer, but this wasn't about me.

Although daily texts of love and support filled with emojis flew back and forth between us for that month of the last two, the word 'death' was never spoken or written between us. Liz remained determined for a miracle cure and I tussled with my heart and mind to allow her the dignity to choose her own way to live her life before she left this world.

The last time I visited her at home, the day before

she was admitted to the hospital, Liz whispered haltingly through light puffs of breath that she would never give up hope. And I nodded through my tears, knowing that the conversations I imagined us having were not going to happen. But then, to my surprise, I felt my body relax for the first time in a year. My hope that we would talk about dying was my wish, not hers, and I finally had to let it go.

The day after that visit, and less than two weeks before Liz died, her oncologist told her that she would have to come off the oral chemotherapy because the cancer was progressing rapidly. There was no more treatment she could offer Liz. The following day Liz told Doug that she had to go to hospital, as she didn't feel able to cope at home. One week later she was transferred to the hospice where she would spend five nights before she died.

The room at the hospice was packed with visitors when I arrived. I approached the bed and Liz's eyes opened.

'Ah, there you are,' she said, with a welcome that felt like a warm homecoming. 'How are you?'

'Happy to see you looking so comfy and settled,' I replied.

'Mmm. Am I not the luckiest woman in the world?'

'What do you mean?' I asked.

'Look around. There's so much love in this room.

I am so lucky.' Liz tried to smile under the oxygen tubing that was inserted into her nostrils.

I looked around at the huge circle of people and saw Doug in an armchair next to Liz's brother-in-law Gerald; Jacqueline and her boyfriend were beside them; Will and his girlfriend held hands; two old friends from Whistler whom I had heard about and recognised from photographs were tucked into the couch under a blanket; two Callanish friends, one playing guitar softly, were sitting on chairs close to the bed; and in a corner on a pillow under the bed was Joey, their spaniel, sleeping. Flowers and cards covered every surface, and photographs were taped to the walls. The room was humming with life.

'I see what you mean,' I said. 'You are pretty lucky.'

Dear, dear Lizzy, I thought, as I covered the deep red roses and the white cosmos with her ashes. People stepped forward in twos and threes to release her ashes to the mandala, until the last person had done so. Finally, large baskets of petals were passed around once more and strewn across the ashes, until the bright colours returned once again, boldly.

'Due Tramonte', meaning 'two sunsets', written by the Italian composer Ludovico Einaudi, was one of Liz's favourite piano pieces, and as fifty of us sat together with the completed mandala at our feet the music rippled across the room, played by Maryliz.

Doug then stepped forward and with a small straw brush slowly and methodically swept the circle of flowers and ash into a large pile in the centre of the canvas, just as I had seen the Tibetan monks do with their mandala at the Museum of Anthropology. The room was silent except for the scratching sound of the brush on the canvas. With the gentle dismantling of the creation, I was aware of the passage of time and the truth about impermanence. My father's favourite saying was 'Everything passes'.

Doug then called on his two children to fold the corners of the canvas together so that they could more easily carry the bundle outside to the creek. A procession of fifty people walked behind the family to the bridge where Maureen, our friend and Cree elder, smudged the bundle with sage smoke and said a prayer to the Creator to keep Liz safe in the natural world that would now become her home.

Doug, Will, Jacqueline and I then clambered down the riverbank to where the water was rushing over several broad tree roots that crossed the width of the creek. I could feel the strength and steadiness of the two red cedars on either side of us as Doug took off his socks and shoes and waded into the pool created by the tree roots to the ledge above a small waterfall rushing down into a larger pool below. He carefully unfolded the canvas bag.

Several feet below us, the group had gathered along the creek bank beside the large pool of crystal-clear water from the Cascade Mountains. I noticed that many were holding hands or had linked arms, and their faces were soft and beautiful. With the help of Jacqueline and Will, Doug opened the bag and slowly poured the petals and the ashes over the tree-root ledge.

Some ashes settled on top of smooth round river rocks, where they shimmered in the late afternoon summer sun, and the petals rushed over the ledge, down the waterfall to the pool below, where the current shaped them into a wide crescent, almost touching the banks on either side. The circle of brightly coloured petals seemed to be held suspended for several minutes before the gentle current of the pool slowly re-shaped them into a column that carried them downstream, finally rounding the bend and disappearing from sight. A few petals were left behind, lodged between stones along the banks. They would likely rest a while before eventually surrendering to the flow of water, perhaps under the darkness of night, lit only by the sliver of a new moon.

Meandering down the path, arm-in-arm, to the feast that awaited us, Doug said with a steadiness to his voice, 'When we can bathe our grief with beauty, everything feels easier.'

And when I think of Liz in the months since her ceremony, I think of her there, in the beautiful creek she loved so much, covered in a mountain of flowers.

Acknowledgements

It took a village to write this book and this is my thank you to many of the villagers who helped me along the way these past eight years. First and foremost, I give thanks to the people in these stories who, despite difficult diagnoses, chose to open to life as best they could. Through them I was shown a roadmap for how to die whole, having fully experienced life. This book is their legacy. May the wisdom in these stories benefit many.

I am indebted to the grieving families of these remarkable people, who bravely read these stories and supported them being sent out into the world. They understand that death is not the end of a relationship and that the love never changes.

When I began writing this book I knew very little about the craft of writing. Many teachers have shown me the way: Betsy Warland, Brian Payton and The

Writer's Studio at Simon Fraser University; my dedicated *non-fictionistas* writing group, especially Karen Lee,
who has been with me every step of the way; Isabel
Huggan at the Humber School for Writers, whose brilliant and incisive critiques humbled and strengthened
me; Pam Houston at Writing By Writers for her review
of my early manuscript and her encouragement to keep
writing; Brooke Warner and Jay Schaefer, who brought
my manuscript up a notch with their skilful editing;
Toby Symington and the Lloyd Symington Foundation
for awarding me a grant to support the writing of this
book; and last, but not least, my Callanish Writes group
of twelve years, who write their way through lives affected
by cancer with such candour.

My heartfelt thanks to James Spackman, my go-to
person for every literary question I have, who introduced
me to my extraordinarily smart and savvy agent Jason
Bartholomew of the bks Agency, London – massive thank
you, Jason. To Hannah Knowles, my brilliant editor
who took my book to the Canongate team with such
respect – thank you, Hannah, for your kind and reas-
suring presence at every turn. To the entire team at
Canongate, especially Jamie Byng, for taking a risk on
an unknown author, Lucy Zhou, my fearless publicist
who tried hard to rescue disappearing media while the
UK locked down at the start of the pandemic, Rafaela
Romaya for her beautiful cover design with the artwork